KETO SLOW COOKER COOKBOOK

Easy to Make Ketogenic Diet Recipes. Turn Your Body Into A Fat-Burning Machine and Lose Weight Fast Using "Low Carb" and Healthy Lifestyle Principles

© Copyright 2020 - All rights reserved.

The content contained within this book may not be reproduced, duplicated or transmitted without direct written permission from the author or the publisher. Under no circumstances will any blame or legal responsibility be held against the publisher, or author, for any damages, reparation, or monetary loss due to the information contained within this book. Either directly or indirectly.

Legal Notice:

This book is copyright protected. This book is only for personal use. You cannot amend, distribute, sell, use, quote or paraphrase any part, or the content within this book, without the consent of the author or publisher.

Disclaimer Notice:

Please note the information contained within this document is for educational and entertainment purposes only. All effort has been executed to present accurate, up to date, and reliable, complete information. No warranties of any kind are declared or implied. Readers acknowledge that the author is not engaging in the rendering of legal, financial, medical or professional advice. The content within this book has been derived from various sources. Please consult a licensed professional before attempting any techniques outlined in this book.

By reading this document, the reader agrees that under no circumstances is the author responsible for any losses, direct or indirect, which are incurred as a result of the use of information contained within this document, including, but not limited to, errors, omissions, or inaccuracies.

KETO SLOW COOKER COOKBOOK

TABLE OF CONTENTS

INTRODUCTION	6
CHAPTER 1: KETOGENIC DIET AND ITS BENEFITS	10
CHAPTER 2: WHAT A SLOW COOKER IS AND HOW IT WORKS	16
CHAPTER 3: BEST PRACTICE TO USE THE SLOW COOKER	20
CHAPTER 4: WHAT CAN YOU EAT AND WHAT SHOULD YOU AVOID	24
CHAPTER 5: HOW TO LOSE WEIGHT ON KETO WITH A SLOW COOKER	28
CHAPTER 6: SHOPPING LIST	32
CHAPTER 7: BREAKFAST RECIPES	36
1. Vanilla Pancakes	37
2. Veggie Turkey Smash	38
3. Paprika Shrimp	39
4. Breakfast Pizza	40
5. Breakfast Sweet Pepper Hash	41
6. Pork Breakfast Sausages	42
7. Potato Breakfast Mix	43
8. Breakfast Veggie Casserole	44
9. Cheddar Jalapeno Breakfast Sausages	45
10. Breakfast Veggie Salad	46
11. Breakfast Pork and Avocado Mix	47
CHAPTER 8: LUNCH RECIPES	**48**
12. Lime Chicken with Savoy Cabbage	49
13. Middle Eastern Lamb Zucchini Casserole	50
14. Ginger Steak Broccoli	51
15. BLT Chicken Salad	52
16. Figs and Goat Cheese-Stuffed Chicken	53
17. Carne Asada	54
18. Amazing Pulled Pork	55
19. Braised Pork Belly	56
20. Peppercorn Short Ribs	57
21. Spicy Italian Sausage and Zucchini Noodles	58
22. Meaty Cauliflower Lasagna	59
23. Chili Verde	60
24. Tandoori Salmon with Fresh Cucumber Salad	61
CHAPTER 9: SNACK RECIPES	**62**
25. Chicken Bites	63
26. Paprika Almonds	63
27. Mixed Nuts	64
28. Beef and Zucchini Wraps	65
29. Cauliflower Bites	66
30. Mushroom Skewers	67
31. Cheese Sticks	68
32. Eggplant Bread	69
33. Almond Granola	70
34. Chili Walnuts	71
35. Pork Bites	72
36. Turkey Meatballs	73

- 37. Tomato Salmon Meatballs 74
- 38. Pecans Bowls 75
- 39. Sausage Dip 76
- 40. Butter Pork Ribs 77
- 41. Chicken Dip 78

CHAPTER 10: DINNER RECIPES 80
- 42. Paprika Pork Tenderloin 81
- 43. Pork Carnitas 82
- 44. Lemongrass Coconut Pulled Pork 83
- 45. Cheesy Cauliflower Gratin 84
- 46. Creamy Ricotta Spaghetti Squash 85
- 47. Creamy Keto Mash 86
- 48. Moist and Spicy Pulled Chicken Breast 87
- 49. Whole Roasted Chicken 88
- 50. Pot Roast Beef Brisket 89
- 51. Seriously Delicious Lamb Roast 90
- 52. Lamb Provençal 91

CHAPTER 11: SIDE DISH RECIPES 92
- 53. Cabbage Steaks 93
- 54. Mashed Cauliflower 94
- 55. Bacon-Wrapped Cauliflower 95
- 56. Cauliflower Casserole 96
- 57. Cauliflower Rice 97
- 58. Curry Cauliflower 98
- 59. Garlic Cauliflower Steaks 99
- 60. Zucchini Gratin 100
- 61. Eggplant Gratin 101
- 62. Moroccan Eggplant Mash 102
- 63. Sautéed Bell Peppers 103
- 64. Garlic Artichoke 104
- 65. Broccoli Stew 105

CHAPTER 12: DESSERT RECIPES 106
- 66. Tapioca and Chia Pudding 107
- 67. Chocolate and Liquor Cream 108
- 68. Dates and Rice Pudding 109
- 69. Butternut Squash Sweet Mix 110
- 70. Almonds, Walnuts, and Mango Bowls 111
- 71. Tapioca Pudding 112
- 72. Berries Salad 113
- 73. Fresh Cream Mix 114
- 74. Pears and Apples Bowls 115
- 75. Pears and Wine Sauce 116
- 76. Creamy Rhubarb and Plums Bowls 117
- 77. Pears and Grape Sauce 118
- 78. Greek Cream Cheese Pudding 119
- 79. Rice Pudding 120
- 80. Greek Cream 121

CHAPTER 13: 7 DAY MEAL PLAN 122
CONCLUSION 124

Introduction

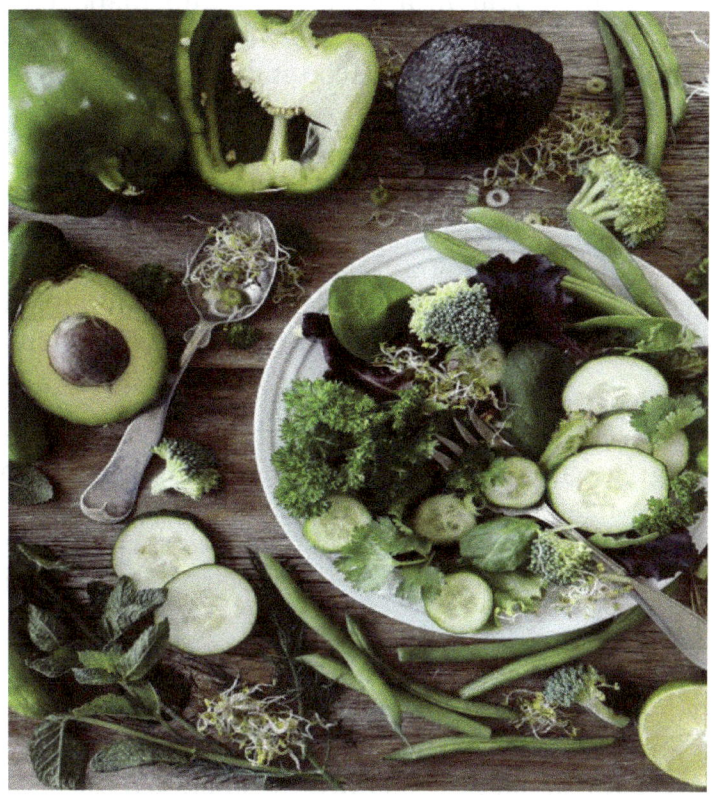

Low-carb diets and the keto diet have been around for some time now, but as we've said, these two diets are different from each other. The effects they have on the body vary too; thus, you should know which type of diet you're following so you know what foods to eat and avoid.

A low-carb diet involves eating minimal amounts of carbohydrates. The dose may differ from one diet to another. Still, the trouble with low-carb diets is that they don't consider the other types of macronutrients, such as proteins and fats. Conversely, the keto diet feels all the macronutrients in the equation, giving your body an alternative fuel source: the ketones. The great thing about the keto diet is that you can measure your ketosis state, unlike the other low-carb diets. This factor allows you to know if the diet is working.

Keto as the Best Diet Plan Out There

There are undoubtedly many weight loss plans obtainable on the market, and it'd be too arrogant to say that the keto weight loss plan is the best among them all. However, it would be fair to mention that the keto eating regimen is a high-quality one for you if it serves your wishes and your goals effectively.

The keto food plan is a low-carb diet designed to place the human body into a heightened ketogenic state, resulting in higher pronounced fat burn and weight loss. It is a reasonably accessible food regimen with various keto-friendly meals readily available in marketplaces at low prices. It isn't an eating regimen that is reserved only for the affluent and elite.

There is no denying how impactful a Keto eating regimen maybe for someone who wants to lose a drastic quantity of weight in a wholesome and managed manner. The keto weight-reduction plan enforces discipline and precision by incorporating macro counting and meal journaling to ensure accuracy and accountability in the weight-reduction project

Food Prep Using Slow Cooker

When it comes to dieting, some cooking methods are more suitable than others, e.g., grilling against frying. However, since Keto cooking is mostly about fats and then protein, you ideally want to try a convenient method that lets you preserve your meals' nutritional goodness and, of course, the necessary fats. And this where slow cooking can come to the rescue. In particular, slow cooking has the following advantages when being on Keto, and you better try this out:

It helps you control what goes inside and precisely the number of sugars and carbs. Since you will choose the ingredients to add, there will be no more guessing or reading food labels to add low or zero sugar and carb ingredients like those listed earlier. It is perhaps the main benefit of using a slow cooker when on Keto. We have made this more comfortable for you in this guide by outlining each recipe's basic nutritional info, so you know what goes inside.

It maintains all the fats inside. By now, you have already realized that fats should be your main priority when on Keto. The issue with other cooking methods is that they dissolve and sometimes burn and evaporate the fat, e.g., grilling, which eliminates the extra fat we need for Keto and makes the fat oxidize isn't healthy at all. On the contrary, slow cooking is one of the very few cooking methods that help preserve the ingredients' original fat without oxidation, provided that you don't overcook your meals.

It lets you prepare low carb yet fully nutritious liquids and sauces. A Slow Cooker is used to make excellent chicken, beef, fish, and veggie stock, which are nutrient-dense yet contain little to none carbs - and yes, this is what we are looking for when on Keto. You can use any of these stocks afterward as your base to cook healthy and delicious keto meats or veggie meals without having to add carb-heavy sauces on top to add flavor. Slow Cookers work best with a bit of liquid; this kind of stocks and sauces can become your staples.

Provided you use your slow cooker properly - and we'll attempt to outline all the necessary steps and some tips and tricks, there is no reason you shouldn't use your slow cooker when being on Keto.

It will be tough to find people who are not in love with home-cooked food. But with the hectic work schedule of these days, it is tough for a working person to find some time for elaborate cooking. It does not mean working people prefer eating out or depending entirely on packaged foods. They, too, want to enjoy the richness of homemade foods, but their work schedules stop them from cherishing their desire.

Culinary innovations have always brought boons for the people who are obsessed with cooking. The slow cooker is one such cooking medium that has solved the people who remain busy all day and desire to have homemade foods at the end of the day. It is nothing but a specialized electric cooker that was designed to cook slowly. Precisely, it is the electronic slow cooker. There are several benefits of cooking with a slow cooker like it is incredibly economical, the cooked foods are healthy, and it is super easy to cook on the slow cooker. The separate cooking settings enable us to cook different ingredients with specific precision. Most importantly, it is effortless to cook the Ketogenic recipes in the slow cooker. As the pot boils slowly, it is easy for working people to dump the ingredients while leaving for work, and when they return home, they can enjoy the bliss of warm homemade dishes.

CHAPTER 1:

Ketogenic Diet and Its Benefits

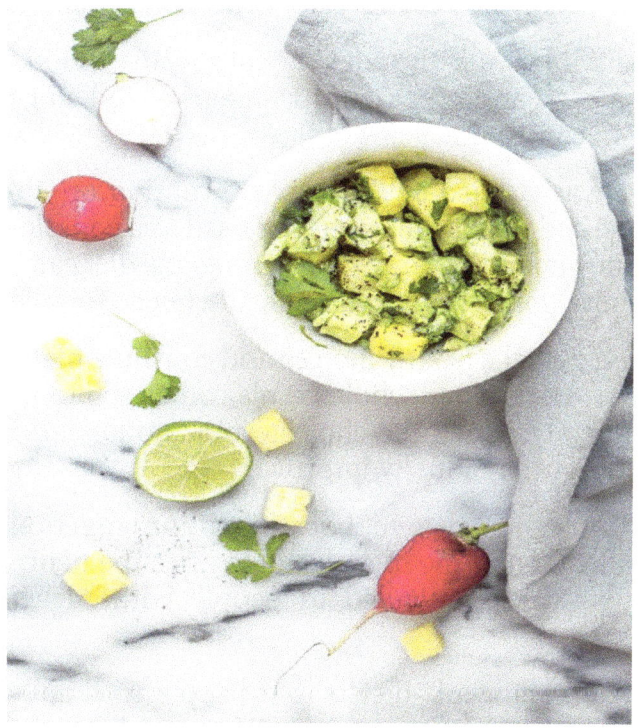

Keto or ketogenic diet is simply a "low carb diet," with a high fat and protein consumption. The Keto diet is often considered to be the same as the Atkin diet. However, they are different. The difference between the two is in the amount of protein consumed.

Another difference is that the keto diet puts the body in ketosis throughout the whole stage. Nevertheless, the Atkin diet only puts the body in ketosis during the first and probably the second phase.

At times, we recommend the ketogenic diet for treating specific ailments. For example, the keto diet can help control diabetes. Also, since the 19th century, the keto diet has been used to treat epilepsy in children.

One of the gaining use of the keto diet is for weight loss. However, there are other low carb diets that you can use for weight loss. Common examples of such diets are South Beach, Dukan, and Paleo diets. What makes the keto diet stands out is fat composition, which is usually between 55-60%.

The word keto is derived from ketosis, which is a natural metabolic process. In other words, we can say that a Ketogenic diet is that combination of meal which can induce or accelerate the rate of ketosis occurring in the human body. The next argument would be why ketosis is considered healthy? Ketosis is the process in which fats are broken down to release energy and ketones. It benefits by producing a fair amount of energy, reducing the body's stored fats, and providing ketones for body metabolism. It is noteworthy that ketosis cannot occur in freely available glucose or Carbohydrates: in the body. Our usual diet contains more carbohydrates than fats; we naturally rely on carbohydrates to extract the required energy. The ketogenic diet is the way of shifting our carb driven body to a fat driven one. Doing so restricts the daily carb intake to 50grams and recommends a fair use of fats instead. All high carbohydrates ingredients are forbidden in this diet plan.

Less sugar intake means lowering the toxic agents in the blood. The same toxins are responsible for causing acne and other skin problems. The ketogenic diet is, therefore, proving to be effective in controlling acne.

When a ketogenic diet was studied to find any prevention or cure for certain types of cancer, the studies suggested that it can indeed be used as a complementary treatment for people who are on chemo and radiotherapy. The ketogenic diet can increase the cancerous cells' oxidative stress more than the normal cells, and hence they can be easily destroyed.

When the ketogenic dieters make health choices and consume high and good fats, contain high-density lipoprotein- HDL. These cholesterols can attach to the bad cholesterol and then removed from the body. When the cholesterol is no longer deposited in the blood vessel, the heart condition will gradually improve.

This high-fat diet is most effective in boosting brain functioning. As the fats are nourishing for the brain cells and the diet also detoxifies the neurons. This factor is why a ketogenic diet is highly recommended to people with Alzheimer's, Epilepsy, and memory loss.

One added advantage of a ketogenic diet is that people with epilepsy can control their seizures. PCOS or Polycystic ovarian syndrome is a medical condition that can bring adverse health effects to a woman. And it is a known fact that a high carb diet further aggravates this condition's damaging effects. Therefore, a ketogenic diet can be used to counter those effects.

The ketogenic diet focuses on reducing your carbohydrate consumption while promoting high fat intake—protein consumption in moderation. The extreme restriction it puts on the carbohydrate consumption may make the ketogenic diet seem like a carb-restrictive diet, but that's not the case. The actual goal of this diet is to encourage a state called "ketosis." Ketosis occurs when the body starts using fats as a primary source of fuel instead of using glucose. Fats are then metabolized for producing ketones. Ketosis happens when your body doesn't have enough glucose.

Glucose is known to create an instant high in the body, followed by a sudden crash. This results in a high level of functioning in the brain, followed by a sudden decline. That's why people who consume high-fat diets experience frequent brain fogs, which hinder their capacity to concentrate on a particular subject. On the other hand, the ketone bodies offer a constant supply of energy without causing any disruption. This is especially beneficial for tissues like the heart and the brain.

The keto diet has become so popular in recent years because of the success people have noticed. Not only have they managed to lose weight, but scientific studies show that the keto diet can help you improve your health in many others. As when starting any new diet or exercise routine, there may seem to be some disadvantages, so we will go over those for the keto diet. But most people agree that the benefits outweigh the adjustment period!

Helps You Lose Weight

For most people, this is the first and foremost benefit of switching to keto! Their former diet method may have stalled for them, or they were starting to notice weight creeping back on. With keto, studies have shown that people have been able to follow this diet and relay fewer hunger pangs and suppressed appetite while losing weight at the same time! You are minimizing your carbohydrate intake, which means less blood sugar spikes. Those fluctuations in blood sugar levels often make you feel hungrier and prone to snacking in between meals. Instead, by guiding the body towards ketosis, you eat a more fulfilling diet of fat and protein and harnessing energy from ketone molecules instead of glucose. Studies show that low carb diets effectively reduce visceral fat (the type of fat you commonly see around the abdomen that increases as you become overweight and obese). This reduces your risk of obesity and improves your health in the long run.

Decreases Risk Of Type 2 Diabetes

The problem with carbohydrates is how unstable they make blood sugar levels. This can be dangerous for people who have diabetes or are considered pre-diabetic due to varying blood sugar levels or family history. Keto is an excellent option because of the minimal intake of carbohydrates it requires. Instead, you are harnessing most of your calories from fat or protein, which will not cause blood sugar spikes and ultimately put less pressure on the pancreas to secrete insulin. Many studies have found that diabetes patients who followed the keto diet lost more weight and eventually reduced their fasting glucose levels. This is excellent news for patients who have unstable blood sugar levels or hope to avoid or reduce their diabetes medication intake.

Improve Cardiovascular Risk Symptoms To Overall Lower Your Chances Of Having Heart Disease

Most people assume that following a keto that is so high in fat content increases your risk of coronary heart disease or heart attack. But the research proves otherwise! Research shows that switching to keto can lower your blood pressure, increase your HDL good cholesterol, and reduce your triglyceride fatty acid levels. That's because the fats you consume on keto are healthy and high-quality fats, which tends to reverse many unhealthy symptoms of heart disease and boost your "good" HDL cholesterol numbers and decrease your "bad" LDL cholesterol numbers. It also reduces the level of triglyceride fatty acids in the bloodstream. A high level of these can lead to stroke, heart attack, or premature death. And what are the high levels of fatty acids linked? Increased consumption of carbohydrates. With the keto diet, you are drastically cutting your carbohydrates intake to improve fatty acid levels and improve other risk factors. A 2018 study on the keto diet found that it can improve as many as 22 out of 26 risk factors for cardiovascular heart disease! These factors can be crucial to some people, especially those with a history of heart disease in their family.

Increase Our Body Energy Levels

We compared the glucose molecules' difference synthesized from a high carbohydrate intake versus ketones produced on the keto diet. Ketones are produced by the liver and use fat molecules you already have stored. This makes them much more energy-rich and an endless fuel source than glucose, a simple sugar molecule. These ketones can physically and mentally give you a burst of energy, allowing you to have greater focus, clarity, and attention to detail.

Decreases Inflammation In The Body

Inflammation on its own is a natural response by the body's immune system, but when it becomes uncontrollable, it can lead to an array of health problems, some severe, some minor.

The many health concerns include acne, autoimmune conditions, arthritis, psoriasis, irritable bowel syndrome, and even acne and eczema. Often, removing sugars and carbohydrates from your diet can help patients of these diseases avoid flare-ups - and the good news is keto does just that! A 2008 research study found that keto decreased a blood marker linked to high body inflammation by nearly 40%. This is excellent news for people who may suffer from inflammatory disease and are willing to change their diet to see improvement hopefully.

Increases Your Mental Functioning Level

Like we elaborated earlier, energy-rich ketones can boost the body's physical and mental levels of alertness.

Research has shown that keto is a much better energy source for the brain than simple sugar glucose molecules are. With nearly 75% of your diet coming from healthy fats, the brain's neural cells and mitochondria have a better energy source to function at the highest level. Some studies have tested patients on the keto diet and found they had higher cognitive functioning, better memory recall, and less memory loss. The keto diet can even decrease the occurrence of migraines, which can be very detrimental to patients.

Decreases Risk Of Diseases Like Alzheimer's, Parkinson's, And Epilepsy.

The keto diet was created in the 1920s as a way to combat Epilepsy in children. From there, research has found that keto can improve your cognitive functioning level and protect brain cells from injury or damage. This discovery reduces neurodegenerative disease risk, which begins in the brain due to neural cells mutating and functioning with damaged parts or lower than peak optimal functioning. Studies have found that the following keto can improve patients' mental functioning who suffer from Alzheimer's or Parkinson's.

These neurodegenerative diseases sadly have no cure, but the keto diet could improve symptoms as they progress. Researchers believe that is due to cutting out carbs from your diet, which reduces blood sugar spikes that the body's neural cells have to adjust continually.

Can Regulate Hormones In Women Who Have Pcos And Pms

Women who have PCOS (polycystic ovary syndrome) have infertility, which can be heartbreaking for young couples trying to start a family. There is no cure for this condition, but it is believed to be related to many similar diabetic symptoms like obesity and high insulin levels. This causes the body to produce more sex hormones, which can lead to infertility. The keto diet has become a popular method to regulate insulin and hormone levels and increase women's chances of getting pregnant.

CHAPTER 2:

What a Slow Cooker is and How it Works

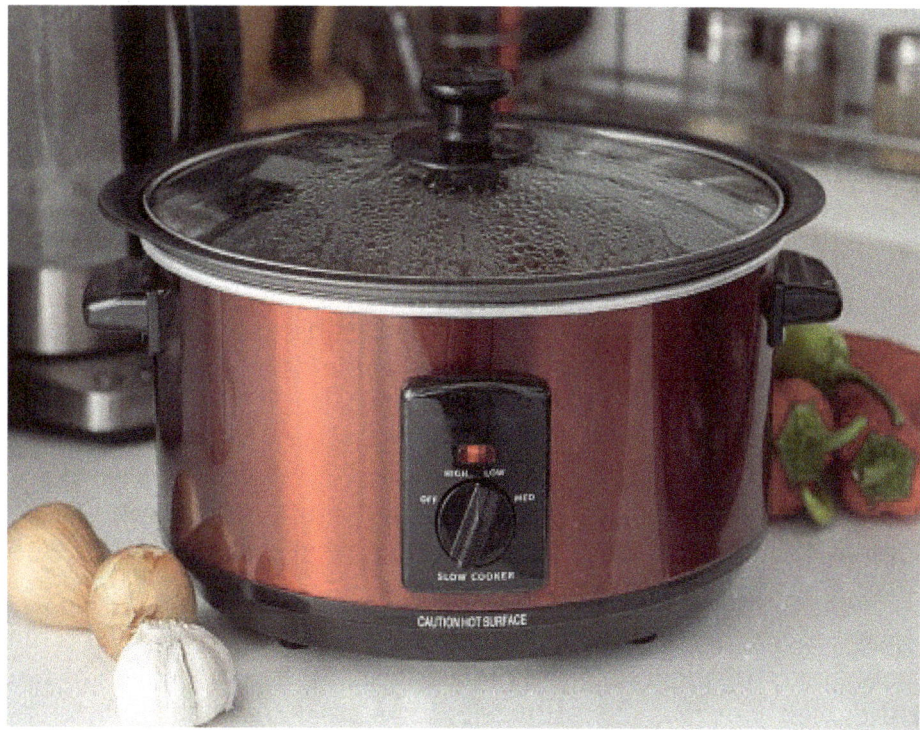

Having a slow cooker is an effortless, fast, and most flexible cooking method at any home. It didn't require you any cooking skills; it saves your time as the slow cooker does all the working time for you, truly safe and can even be used in any places like a hotel room or even student dorm as they possess a kettle like-shape, making it more portable than a stove. In the following guides, we will discuss some of the helpful basic ways to guarantee that you get the best out of your slow cooker.

What Is It?

The slow cooker appeared in 1970 and was marketed as a bean cooker. But as modified, people started to use it to heat food and keep it warm for prolonged periods. And look how far we've come; people are cooking delicious healthy meals in it. It is a perfect small kitchen appliance consisting of a glass lid, porcelain, or a ceramic pot (inside the heating unit) and a heating element. The modern Slow Cooker could be of an oval or round shape and various sizes, from small to large. The Slow Cookers have two settings: LOW (it corresponds to the temperature of 200°F mostly) and HIGH (up to 300°F). The WARM selection among most Slow cookers' options nowadays allows keeping the prepared dishes warm for a long time. Some of the Slow Cooker models have a timer that will enable you to control cooking time if you are busy.

Why, Slow Cook?

Some of the reasons to use a slow cooker include:

- **Enhances flavor:** Cooking ingredients over several hours with spices, herbs, and other seasonings creates vegetables and proteins that burst with delicious flavors. This slow process allows the flavors to mellow and deepens for an enhanced eating experience.

- **Saves time:** Cooking at home takes a great deal of time: prepping, sautéing, stirring, turning the heat up and down, and watching the meal so that it does not over- or undercook. If you're unable to invest the time, you might find yourself reaching convenience foods instead of healthy choices. Slow cookers allow you to do other activities while the meal cooks. You can put your ingredients in the slow cooker in the morning and come home to a perfectly cooked meal.

- **Convenient:** Besides the time-saving aspect, using a slow cooker can free up the stove and other dishes. This can be very convenient for large holiday meals or when you want to serve a side dish and entrée and a delectable dessert. Clean up is simple when you use the slow cooker for messy meals because most inserts are non-stick or are easily cleaned with a little soapy water. Each meal is prepared in either just the machine or using one additional vessel to sauté ingredients. There is no wide assortment of pots, pans, and baking dishes to contend with at the end of the day.

- **Low heat production:** If you have ever cooked dinner on a scorching summer afternoon, you will appreciate the short amount of heat produced by a slow cooker. Even after eight hours of operation, slow cookers do not heat your kitchen, and you will not be sweating over the hot stovetop. Slow cookers use about a third of conventional cooking methods, just a little more energy than a traditional light bulb.

- **Supports healthy eating:** Cooking your food at high heat can reduce the nutrition profile of your foods, breaking down and removing the majority of vitamins, minerals, and antioxidants while producing harmful chemical compounds that can contribute to disease. Low-heat cooking retains all the goodness that you want for your diet.

- **Saves Money:** Slow cookers save you money because of the low amount of electricity they use. The best ingredients for slow cooking are the less expensive cuts of beef and heartier inexpensive vegetables. Tougher cuts of meat—brisket, chuck, shanks—break down beautifully to fork-tender goodness. Another cost-saving benefit is that most 6-quart slow cookers will produce enough of a recipe to stretch your meals over at least two days. Leftovers are one of the best methods for saving money.

The Right Cooker For You

Slow cookers have changed a lot over the years. These days you can purchase models that range from straightforward models to ones that look like they should be on a space station. When buying the right model for your needs, you have to consider what you are cooking, how many portions, and if you will be home during the cooking process. All these factors are essential when deciding on your slow cooker's size, shape, and features.

Size and Shape

Slow cookers come in many sizes and shapes, so it is essential to consider your needs and what will work best for the food prepared on the keto diet. Some models range from ½-quart to large 8-quart models and everything in-between.

The small slow cookers (½-quart to 2-quart) are usually used for dips or sauces and recipes designed for one person. Medium-sized slow cookers (3-quart to 4-quart) are great for baking or meals that create food for two to three people. The slow cooker recommended for most of the recipes in this book is the 5-quart to 6-quart model because it is perfect for the massive cuts of meat on the keto diet and can prepare food for four people, including leftovers. The enormous 7-quart to 8-quart appliance is meant for huge meals. If you have money in your budget, owning both a 3-quart and 6-quart model would be the best of both worlds.

When it comes to shapes, you will have to decide between round, oval, and rectangular. Round slow cookers are fine for stews and chili but do not work well for large meat pieces. These should probably not be your choice. Oval and rectangular slow cookers allow for the ingredients you will regularly use that are large, like roasts, ribs, and chops, and have the added advantage of fitting loaf pans, ramekins, and casserole dishes, as well. Some desserts and bread are best cooked in another container placed in the slow cooker, and you will see several recipes in this book that use that technique.

Features

Now that you know the recommended slow cooker's size and shape, it is time to consider what you want this appliance to do for you. Depending on your budget, at a minimum, you want a slow cooker with temperature controls that cover warm, low, and high, as well as a removable insert. These are the primary features of the bare-bones models that will get the job done. However, suppose you want to truly experience a set-it-and-forget-it appliance that creates the best meals possible in this cooking environment. In that case, you might want to consider the following features:

- **Digital programmable controls:** You can program temperature, when the slow cooker starts, how long it cooks, and when the slow cooker switches to warm.

- **Glass lid:** These are heavier and allow you to look into the slow cooker without removing them, so there is little heat loss. Opt for a cap with clamps, and you can transport your cooked meal easily to parties and gatherings if needed.

- **Temperature probe:** Once you have a slow cooker with this feature, you will wonder how you cooked previously without it. The temperature probe allows you to cook your meat, poultry, and egg dishes to an exact temperature and then switches to warm when completed.

- **Precooking feature:** Some models have a precooking feature that allows you to brown your meat and poultry right in the insert. You will still have to take the time to do this step, but you won't have a skillet to clean afterward.

CHAPTER 3:

Best Practice To Use The Slow Cooker

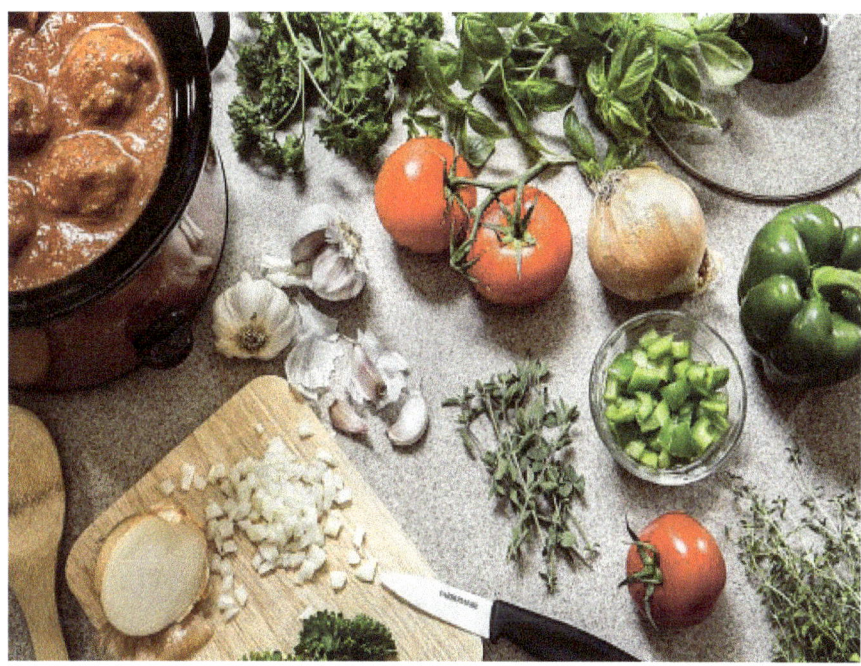

Tips for Using Slow Cookers

Knowing how to use a slow cooker best can be a game-changer in terms of simplifying your life. Here are a few tips that can make using your slow cooker an even more satisfying experience.

1. Meal plan and pre-prep your food as much as possible. Indeed, sometimes you can just throw random ingredients into a slow cooker and turn out a masterpiece. It is also true that sometimes that philosophy can result in a culinary disaster. I know that you are probably busy, and meal planning may or may not be on your priority list. However, you should try to give a little thought to what you might like to cook during the week. Taking a short time at the beginning of the week can save you significant time over the week if you prepare a particular dish or use specific ingredients, pre-wash, or cut them in advance to save yourself later. This is especially helpful if you are assembling a slow cooker full of goodness in the morning before you rush out the door.

2. To make your slow cooker meal a no-fuss event, prepare everything the night before. You can brown meat, cut vegetables, and assemble everything in the evening. Once it is built, place it in the refrigerator, grab it and get it going in the morning.

3. In most cases, slow cooker times can be adjusted to suit your schedule. The recipes in this book were created using a certain quantity of food at a low temperature to allow the dishes to take eight to ten hours to cook to perfection. If you would like to shorten that cooking time, simply cut back a little on the ingredients and increase the temperature to high. Generally speaking, improving the condition can take two to four hours off the cooking time, depending on the dish.

4. Consider browning the meat. Many of the recipes in this book call for browning the meat or quickly sautéing some vegetables. Do you need to do this step? For that question, the answer is no. However, if you are looking for the highest quality results, then the answer is yes. Browning the meat before you place it in the slow cooker helps maintain the meat's moisture, flavor, and juiciness. When you sauté vegetables, you change the ingredient's character and slightly taste something a little more desirable. Take onions, for instance. You can just place them in the slow cooker, and they will absorb juices and soften during cooking. The result is often delicious. Other times, you might want to sauté them a little to bring out their natural sweetness to a level that slow cooking alone cannot do.

5. When you brown your meat, don't forget to scrape the pan. There is a lot of goodness left in the bottom of a pan used to brown a meat piece. The same is true for the oils or moisture left after sautéing vegetables. Take the extra minute and scrape the pan into the slow cooker to keep all the different flavors.

6. Beware the dairy. If you follow a ketogenic diet, you are likely also enjoying creamy, full-fat dairy products daily. Full-fat dairy is excellent as it provides valuable nutrition and necessary fat calories. You can include full-fat dairy in your slow cooker creations. You have to be a little thought about how you do it. First of all, dairy that sits in the heat all day is going to curdle a bit. It is okay if it is small and mixed with other ingredients to help offset the effect. Sometimes the thickening that happens is just what you are expecting. However, in most cases, when you use more massive amounts of dairy, you will want to add it towards the end of the cooking time, usually in the last hour of cooking. This method will help maintain the texture and integrity of the dairy ingredients. It adds a little bit of time in the end, but it is well worth it.

7. Use the highest quality ingredients you can afford. When someone has a negative slow cooker experience, they used inferior ingredients, and didn't mean you have to break the bank on all grass-fed or organic ingredients. What is does mean is pay attention to where your money is best spent on quality and where you can afford to skimp. Also, cook with ingredients that are in season in your area whenever possible. A tomato that comes from the farmer across town will be far superior to one that traveled a thousand miles just to reach your grocer's shelf.

8. Don't overfill your slow cooker. For best results, your slow cooker should not be more than three-quarters of the way full. It allows plenty of room for the

heat to circulate and cook everything evenly. If you find that your slow cooker is overstuffed, simply cut back on the bulky ingredients a little.

9. Resist the temptation to be lifting the lid and inhaling the savory aroma constantly. Yes, it smells great. However, you are disrupting the cooking process by allowing the heat to escape. Then the slow cooker has to work to get back up to the proper cooking temperature again.

10. Consider the placement of the ingredients in your slow cooker. One of the best features of a slow cooker is the "dump and go" potential. Slow cooker meals are generally low fuss and require little more than tossing the ingredients in and turning it on. There are times, though, when a little forethought about how the elements are placed can make a big difference to the result. The most heat is going to come from the bottom of the device. This means that what you put on the bottom is going to have more surface-to-surface heat. Sometimes, you might want this to be the meat.

11. Cut your ingredients in uniform pieces and keep texture in mind. Raw pumpkin is quite dense and can be cut into smaller, even pieces to ensure they are cooked to tender perfection. Mushrooms, on the other hand, cook relatively quickly and should be added in large chunks, or even in the last hour or two of cooking, if you will be home to add them. Spinach and other greens should be added a short while before serving. When this is possible, give them time to wilt.

12. The meat thermometer is your friend. Even if that roast has been in there for eight hours and it looks delectably done, take a minute and stick a meat thermometer in it. For most meats that are not beef, you want a temperature of 160°F. With meat, you can have a bit more of a range depending upon the doneness you prefer. As a reference, 140°F was considered medium-rare for beef.

13. Your slow cooker not only makes leftovers super easy, but they often taste even better. The slow cooking process gives the ingredients more time together to build up the flavor. If you have bits, refrigerate them overnight and turn the slow cooker back on the next day. Add a little extra liquid if you need to for moisture.

Caring for Your Slow Cooker and Cleaning It

Your slow cooker's instruction manual contains the most pertinent information for caring for your slow cooker. Here are some essential tips:

- Try not to cook longer than the cooking time given in the recipe, so the food doesn't get burned.

- Do not add cold ingredients to a slow cooker that has already been heated. The insert is sensitive and may crack or break.

- Turn off, unplug, and allow your slow cooker to cool down before cleaning.

- The heating base should not be submerged in water or any liquid.
- Always remove the lid first before releasing the insert or stoneware.
- The slow cooker insert is dishwasher safe. When using the dishwasher isn't enough, the following may be used:
  - hot, soapy water
  - baking soda (for gentle scrubbing)
  - vinegar
- Use a slow cooker liner or non-stick cooking spray for easy cleaning after cooking.

Remember these simple tips, and you'll be able to use your slow cooker for many meals and through many happy family occasions!

CHAPTER 4:

What Can You Eat and What Should You Avoid

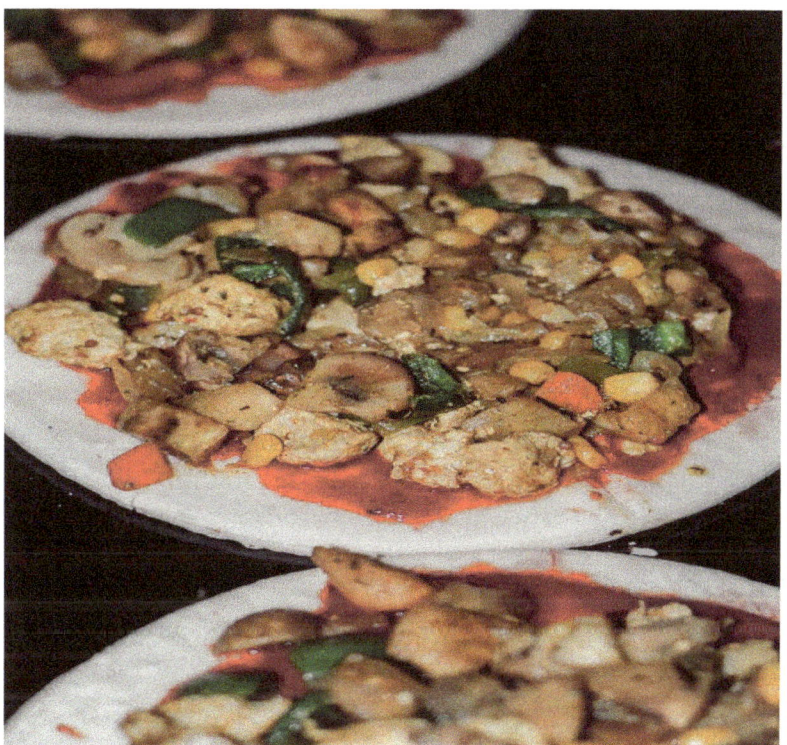

What to Enjoy on this Diet?

- Keto-Friendly Animal Produce

Meat doesn't contain carbohydrates in any form, so it is wholly allowed on a ketogenic diet. It includes seafood, poultry: chicken, turkey, duck, beef, mutton, lamb, pork, etc.

- Low Carb Vegetables

When identifying vegetables as ketogenic, You must keep this simple rule in mind that those grown mostly below the ground are rich in carbohydrates and are not keto-friendly, mostly underground tubers.

Whereas all the vegetables above the ground are keto-friendly, these include green leafy vegetables, tomatoes, cucumber, asparagus, broccoli, cabbage, cauliflower, etc.

- Keto Seeds and Nuts

Seeds and dry nuts do not contain excessive carbohydrates, and a balanced amount of them can be taken on a keto diet. Pumpkin seeds, pistachio, almonds, etc. are all allowed.

- Limited Dairy Items

We need to be a bit more careful about dairy products as not all of them are prohibited on a keto diet. Milk contains more carbohydrates; therefore, it should be avoided. Whereas cheese, yogurt, cream, cream cheese, butter, eggs are all keto-friendly.

Animal milk can be substituted with:

1. Soy milk
2. N Almond milk
3. Coconut milk
4. Macadamia milk
5. Hemp milk

- Keto-Friendly Fruits

Like veggies, not all fruits are suitable for the ketogenic diet. Some are high in carbs like apple, pineapple, banana, etc. However, you can enjoy blackberries, cranberries, avocado, coconut, blueberries, strawberries, as they have low carb content.

- Healthy Fats and Oils

When it comes to fat, there is no compulsion or reservations for a ketogenic diet. You can use all plant oils and animal fat, including olive oil, butter, canola oil, etc.

- Low Carb-Sweeteners

1. Stevia
2. Erythritol
3. Swerve
4. Monk fruit sweetener
5. Natvia

What Should you be Avoiding?

1. Say No to Grains

Edible grains are a great source of carbohydrates, wheat, rice, barley, millet, etc. So, these all are strictly forbidden on a keto-friendly diet. Products obtained from these grains are also not allowed, including wheat flour, all-purpose flour, rice flours, etc.

This kind of flour can be replaced with:

- Almond flour
- Coconut flour

2. Animal Milk

All dairy items are allowed on a ketogenic diet except for animal milk.

3. No Legumes

All legumes are grown underground, and they are high carb food items. Legumes include all lentils, beans, and chickpeas. None of them are keto-friendly and should be avoided entirely.

4. Avoid all Sugars

Sugar is nothing but the purest form of carbohydrates. Hence it should be avoided entirely, whether white sugar, granulated, brown, baking sugar, etc. Products containing a high sugar level are also prohibited like molasses, honey, dates, processed food, and beverages.

5. High Glycaemic Fruits

Fruits like banana, oranges, apples, pomegranate, pineapple, pears, and watermelon are rich in sugar. Avoid using these fruits, especially on a ketogenic diet. Avoid extracts obtained from these fruits

6. Underground Tubers and Starchy Vegetables

Tubers are underground vegetables, and they store food for plants in the form of carbohydrates. These include potatoes, beetroots, and yams. They all are not suitable for a ketogenic diet.

CHAPTER 5:

How to Lose Weight on Keto with a Slow Cooker

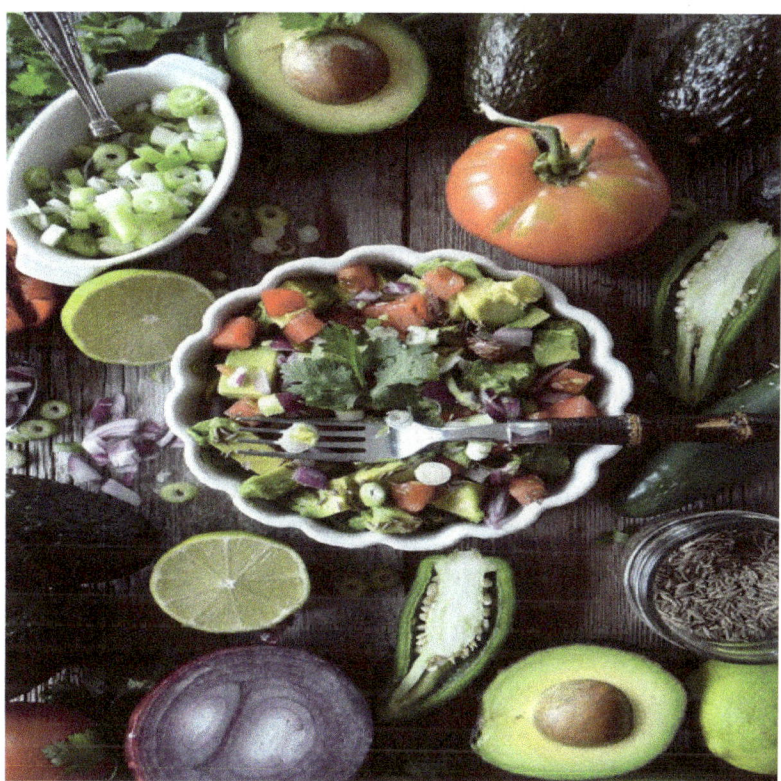

Weight loss is the weight you lose when your body undergoes the experts' term as a caloric deficiency. When your body finds itself in a state where calorie input is lesser than what it needs for daily function, it will seek energy from your body's energy stores. Most of the time, these would be from the stores of glucose found in the liver and your muscle. The other major energy store in our body would be the fats we carry on our frame. This time is when the tricky part comes in. If your body isn't conditioned for burning fats, it will quickly use up the glucose stores, and that is when the feeling of hunger will come in to derail you from your weight loss mission potentially.

Some Common Weight Loss Principles to Note

Keep hunger at bay – Many folks start dieting to lose their excess weight and attempt to get healthy, but quite a number fail and fall by the wayside. In the end, these folks have to resort to medications and drugs to suppress the symptoms and conditions that accompany obesity. It is not a pretty sight. It is sometimes quite depressing to see people consign themselves to such a fate when more efficient and healthier solutions are just around the corner.

They may have started strong and see results after some time, but invariably, the one thing that always put paid to these efforts would be the feeling of hunger that many of these diets entail. Take a straightforward calorie restriction diet plan. For example, if your daily requirement works out to be about 1,750 calories, just polishing off a bagel for a snack would set you back by 250 calories. That is like one-seventh of your total requirement. Imagine eating seven bagels for the whole day. Would that be enough?

The trick is to get onto a diet and lifestyle change to feel full and keep the hunger pangs at bay and get your body to lose weight. Know of any diet that does just that?

Be sustainable – There are many ways to lose weight, that is for sure. Considering the latest fad diet, juicing, fasting, going the vegan way. I have to say that I hold all these methodologies in high esteem, and it is my opinion that each of them has its benefits for the human body.

Fasting, for example, is an excellent way to let the body rebalance itself and to get rid of toxins that have built up over time. One of the side effects of fasting would be a loss of body weight. However, you would not expect a person to fast for a lifetime without consuming food. For any method of efficient weight loss, it must be sustainable in practice to allow for continued shedding of the excess pounds and also to prevent the dreaded bounce back in weight that has plagued so many

One of the benchmarks of sustainability for diets would be the ease of implementing it in everyday life. Imagine if you are on a diet that requires you to eat six to seven small meals a day, you would have to pack for those meals and find the time to consume them during the workday.

Exercise – Regarded as one of the main pillars for weight loss, exercise, especially strength training, can help build muscles that burn more calories, not to mention getting you that ripped figure. Yes, it was always good to dream that some magic pill in the market could get you whipped in shape without any effort, but alas, it remains a dream.

Strength training, done through weights at home or hitting the gym, is one of the surest ways to lose weight. It would be advisable to have a schedule for the days you work out to concentrate on specific muscle groups. This targeted training helps to speed muscle development, leading to higher calorie usage and hence weight loss.

There will be loads of resources online on how to work out a proper strength training routine. The more important thing is to have the discipline to keep plugging at it until you see or feel the results. It will be worth it.

Ketogenic Diet and Weight Loss

Having touched on what weight loss was and the common principles behind it, let us now look at how the ketogenic diet can become one of your staunchest allies in the bulge's battle.

Being mindful of hunger – As we said earlier, keeping hunger pangs at bay is one of the most important ways to ensure your weight loss regime is on track. The keto diet does this precisely by encouraging the consumption of fats, which by nature is more satiating and gives you the feeling of fulfillment and hence stops those frequent trips to the kitchen pantry for more food.

The other spiffy thing about going on the keto diet is the resultant leveling of your insulin levels. Insulin is known to induce the feeling of hunger, and when ketosis kicks in, you no longer have those roller-coaster ups and downs that are associated with the consumption of carbs. This stability means your hunger pangs are mainly held at bay due to your body's insulin reduction.

Now, you will eat when your body truly feels hungry, and that is quite liberating. Not to mention that your weight loss journey will become much more straightforward because of this removal of hunger pangs from the overall equation.

Quicker recovery from exercise – while we engage in strength training in our bid to lose weight and get in shape, our bodies need time to recover from the physical activity. Practitioners of the keto diet will find that their recovery time will be somewhat quicker than others.

The reduction of carbohydrates to be replaced by fats is why body inflammation levels will come down. Once inflammation is down, your muscles tend to recover faster from fatigue, allowing you to put in more sessions due to the shortened recovery period.

The more stable energy levels are achieved due to fewer fluctuations in the blood sugar levels, and a diet switch allows you to work out without feeling faintish or light-headed. Typical hypoglycemia symptoms or just a simple lack of glucose in the bloodstream are burning fats and producing ketones as a more stable energy source!

When compared to more motivation from quicker results to Quick question, which would you prefer? A weight-loss method that requires you to toil consistently at it for up to six months a pop and to have a loss of four or five pounds to show for it, or the ketogenic diet that can see weight loss come in the range of twenty to thirty pounds within six to seven weeks?

If you are like me, then the choice would be the latter. Quicker results, especially in the arena of weight loss, are almost always going to be a welcome morale booster. When you see how much weight you have lost within those short weeks, it gives you confidence that this method works and, you gain that conviction and strength to keep going.

What happens here when you transit over to the keto diet is that you have lowered insulin levels. High insulin tells our kidneys to retain more salt and water, so we have less salt and water retention when the insulin levels decrease. This process leads to a rapid decrease in the number on the weighing scales, but more importantly, the keto diet also provides for a sustained drive in the loss of body weight through the burning of fat stores.

Some Tips for Weight Loss

This list is by no means an exhaustive but just something to let you kick start the weight loss journey if you haven't already. The tips are all quickly actionable and easy to follow, though some may require a little more effort than the other, these are all ideas which have been known to work for people in pursuit of weight loss.

Record what you eat – Get a notebook if you are of the more pen and paper variety, or simply just use the note function in your smartphone to record the food you are consuming throughout the day. This gives you a sense of accountability when you sit down and review what you have eaten at the end of the day. You might be surprised at the amount of food you have taken in, which will serve as a timely reminder to do better the next day.

Get an accountability partner – Many people do better in tasks requiring discipline when required to report to somebody else. Getting an accountability partner will add a sense of responsibility and the desire not to disappoint the partner when you register on your weight loss daily activities. Having someone to persuade and encourage you during this period can also be immensely gratifying, and that could be the added push to keep you on track for the weight loss journey.

Get enough sleep – It is by no means a measure of a surprise to know that lack of sleep hampers your weight loss efforts by the simple increase of the hormone cortisol in our body system. Cortisol increases our appetite and hunger sensations, which is why getting sufficient sleep can do simple wonders in letting you shed excess pounds. You will feel less cranky and more energized too!

Be mindful when eating – We get the feeling of fullness and satiation when we concentrate on the food that we are chewing and not get distracted by the ever-present mobile devices, or the other assorted distractions available in this modern world have our meals. When eating, just eat! I know it is easier said than done, but you can try counting the number of chews for that mouthful of food, get to seven or ten chews before swallowing. It helps to focus your mind on the food you consume, and as a bonus, you are helping your stomach with better digestion!

Avoid processed foods – Yeap, that means the ice-creams, donuts, and creamy cakes have got to take a backseat when it comes to your food selection. Pile on the whole and natural foods because those are nutrient-dense items that will ensure you do not take in empty calories. Most of the processed food found today contain quite a bit of sugar and are pretty much deficient in the nutrients department, hence the term empty calories! The sugar eats into your daily calorie limit while not providing you with the essential nutrients your body needs. Go for chicken meat instead of chicken nuggets, whole potatoes instead of fries. You get the idea. Putting real foods on your platter gives you more bang for the buck in terms of your daily calorie limit, where you ensure that the calories you take in supplies your body with the nutrients that it needs to function well.

CHAPTER 6:

Shopping List

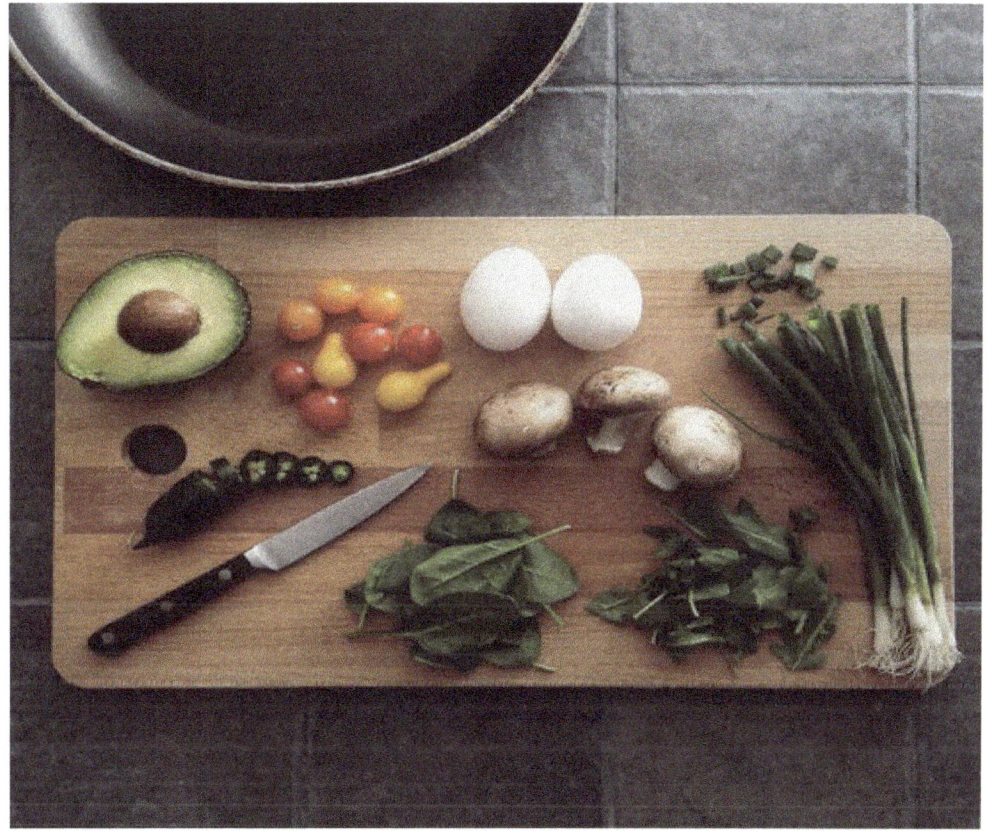

The first step in preparing for a person's first keto shopping trip is to clean out their home—pantry, and fridge, freezer, and all. This process ensures that a person gets rid of any possible food temptation while feeling confident about the diet, helping in crisis moments later down the road.

Knowing what to throw out can be tricky if you are not intimately familiar with the keto diet, but there are some rules of thumb. The first is to eliminate all grains and starches; this means rice, bread, corn, potatoes, and anything else a person might have stored in their pantry. It also includes all alcohol that isn't a dry red wine, oils that do not have healthy fats, margarine, and anything high in sugar or artificial sweeteners. At this stage, it can help look at food labels to know what to toss everything with sugar or ingredients that are hard to pronounce should be discarded.

Throwing away food can be difficult for some people to embrace, but it is essential to remember that this step will get them through to the end. Discarding bad food shows that the person is choosing to do something better for their body, and it should empower them to follow their diet once they get better nutrition in the house.

Once all of the wrong foods have been purged from the house, it is time to restock with the approved foods mentioned earlier in the book. Fatty meats, dairy products, eggs, and low-carb veggies should be plentiful in the home. When composing the grocery list, it is also important to remember the little things such as oils and nuts. These can serve as snacks or the base for delicious dipping sauces to keep meals interesting. Nut butter is also a great thing to have on hand when hunger kicks in unexpectedly.

This makes the best time to embrace the kitchen and stock it with whatever it needs to make cooking easy. Kitchen staples should include a sharp knife, a cutting board, a skillet, pots, pans, mixing bowls, a blender, and a slow cooker or Instant Pot.

When a person's home has been prepared, they can then begin working on their grocery list. It is vital for beginners not to become overwhelmed while compiling the grocery list, even though it will differ from what they are used to. They need to keep in mind the acceptable primary food groups and focus on those instead of all the things they cannot eat.

The first thing to consider is low-carb veggies. These include dark leafy greens such as spinach and arugula, eggplants, tomatoes, broccoli, cauliflower, and anything not too sweet. Vegetables will be the primary source of vitamins and should not be ignored in the keto diet. Also, in the produce department, the few fruits that are low enough in sugar are acceptable on the keto diet. Focusing on berries—strawberries, blueberries, blackberries, raspberries—as well as coconut, lemons, and limes can provide the sweet fix a person might need at the beginning of keto.

The next focus is protein, which can be found in seafood, red meat, chicken, and eggs. For seafood, a person should focus on fatty fish such as salmon, sardines, tuna, shrimp, cod, etc. These are excellent sources of omega-3 fatty acids, which the body can only get from food and help a wide variety of functions and organs. Red meats such as beef, venison, and lamb are all great sources of saturated fats for the keto diet. A person should be sure to grab the fattiest cuts of these meats available to reap the most benefits from them. Chicken with the skin on is another excellent source of leaner, and eggs contain a high amount of fat and protein, making them keto powerhouses.

Other go-to's are typically in the dairy aisle; full-fat cheese, plain Greek yogurt, cream, and butter can all be excellent fat sources and an easy way to add flavor to meals. Almonds, walnuts, macadamia nuts, chia seeds, and others are all quick snacks a person can grab to tide them over in the day. Finally, for cooking, a person should focus on healthy oils such as olive oil, coconut oil, MCT oil, and avocado oil.

Refrigerator Items:

- Non-fat plain yogurt, 0% fat Greek yogurt
- Low-fat almond milk, coconut milk, almond milk
- Fresh fruit (apples, melon, bananas, berries, oranges, grapefruit, pears, peaches, Parmesan cheese, goat cheese, feta cheese

- Eggs
- Thinly-sliced turkey breast for sandwiches and snacks
- Diced or sliced veggies like celery, cucumbers, carrots for dipping
- Meat:
- Fish, shrimp, poultry, beef, pork, lamb
- Canned & Bottled Items:
- Canned beans: black beans, chickpeas, cannellini beans, lentils, red kidney beans
- Tomato paste, canned tomatoes
- Reduced-sodium broths: chicken broth, beef broth, vegetable broth
- Grains & Legumes:
- Whole-wheat flour
- Rolled oats, whole-wheat couscous, brown rice
- Nuts, Seeds & Fruits:
- Almonds, Pecans, Walnuts, Sesame seeds, peanuts
- Natural nut butter: peanut, almond
- Dried fruits: apricots, cherries, cranberries, prunes, figs, dates, raisins
- Oils, Condiments, Vinegar, Flavorings
- Extra-virgin olive oil, canola oil, sunflower oil, almond oil
- Vanilla extract
- Salt, black pepper, Dried Onions, Ginger, Garlic
- Dried herbs: dried thyme leaves, dill, crumbled dried sage, oregano, tarragon,
- Spices: allspice, chili powder, cumin seeds, ground cumin, ground cinnamon, coriander seeds, ground ginger, dry mustard, paprika, crushed red pepper, turmeric

CHAPTER 7:

Breakfast Recipes

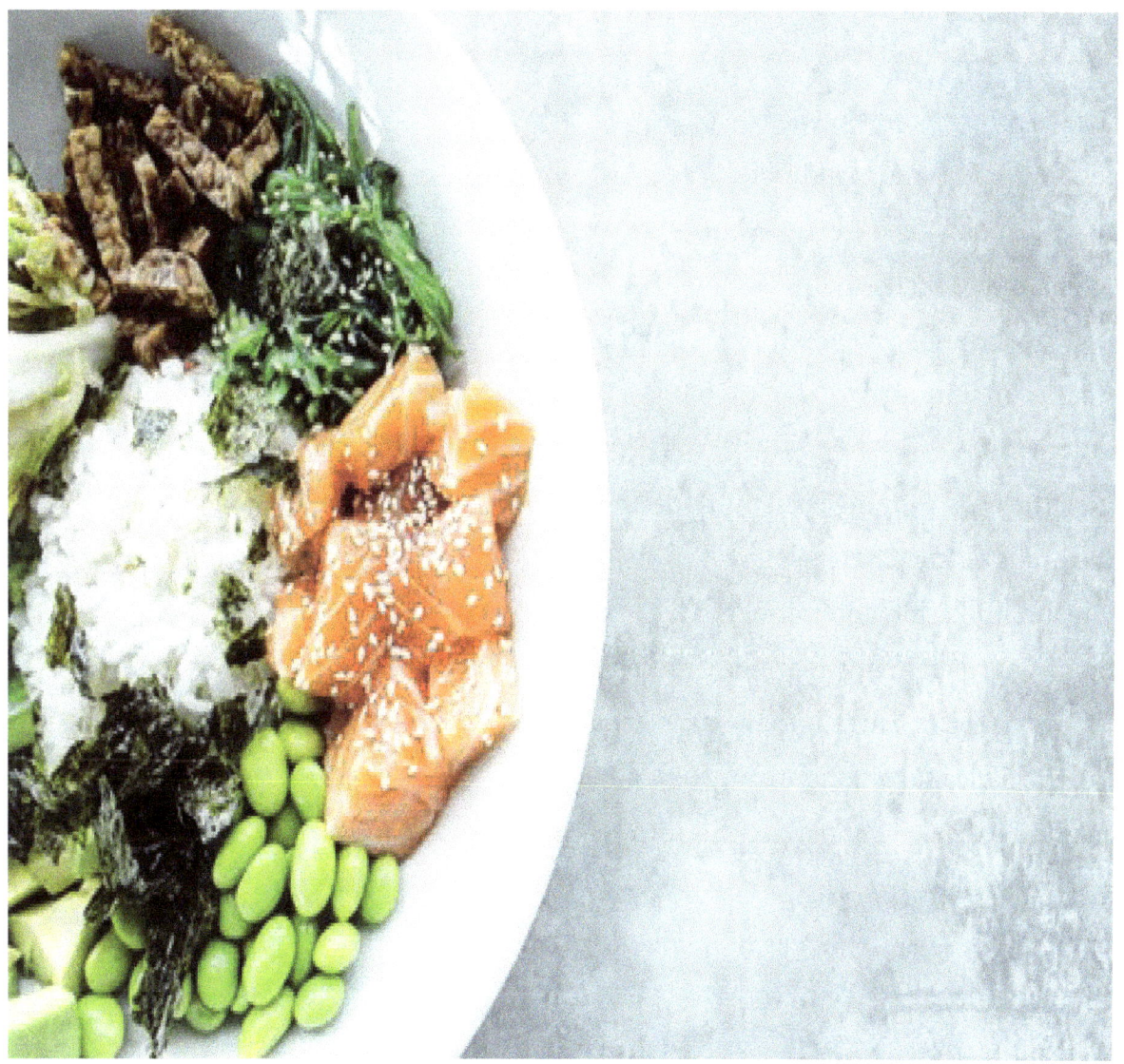

1. Vanilla Pancakes

Preparation Time: 15 minutes

Cooking time: 2 hours

Servings: 6

Ingredients:

1 cup coconut flour

Two eggs, beaten

One teaspoon baking powder

One tablespoon vanilla extract

One tablespoon ghee

½ cup almond milk

¾ teaspoon salt

¼ teaspoon nutmeg

Directions:

Whisk the eggs with the coconut flour and baking powder in the mixing bowl.

Add vanilla extract and ghee.

Then add milk, salt, and nutmeg.

Stir the pancake mixture carefully until smooth.

Pour the pancake batter into the slow cooker and close the lid.

Cook the pancake for 2 hours on High.

When the pancake is cooked, cut it into servings and serve.

Enjoy!

Nutrition: Calories 173, Fat 10.4, Fiber 8.5, Carbs 15.3, Protein 5

2. Veggie Turkey Smash

Preparation Time: 15 minutes

Cooking time: 7 hours

Servings: 4

Ingredients:

One eggplant

One onion

9 oz ground turkey

One green pepper, chopped

One tablespoon butter

One teaspoon chili flakes

Directions:

Peel the eggplant and onion and chop both into small pieces.

Then combine the chopped vegetables with the green pepper.

Add butter, chili flakes, and ground turkey.

Mix and transfer to the slow cooker.

Cook the turkey smash for 7 hours on Low.

When the time is done, stir the cooked meal carefully and transfer to serving bowls.

Enjoy!

Nutrition: Calories 196, Fat 10.2, Fiber 5.2, Carbs 10.7, Protein 19.2

3. Paprika Shrimp

Preparation Time: 10 minutes

Cooking time: 1 hour

Servings: 6

Ingredients:

1-pound shrimp, peeled

¼ teaspoon ground black pepper

One teaspoon paprika

¼ teaspoon minced garlic

¾ cup chicken stock

Directions:

Sprinkle the peeled shrimp with the ground black pepper and paprika.

Then sprinkle the shrimp with the minced garlic and stir well.

Place the chicken stock in the slow cooker.

Add the seasoned shrimp and close the lid.

Cook the shrimp for 1 hour on High.

Then transfer the shrimps to the serving plate and serve!

Nutrition: Calories 92, Fat 1.4, Fiber 0.2, Carbs 1.5, Protein 17.4

4. Breakfast Pizza

Preparation Time: 15 minutes

Cooking time: 3 hours

Servings: 4

Ingredients:

Four tablespoons almond flour

½ teaspoon baking powder

¾ teaspoon salt

Two eggs, beaten

4 oz ham, chopped

One teaspoon Italian seasoning

One teaspoon olive oil

3 oz Parmesan, grated

Directions:

Mix the almond flour and baking powder.

Add salt and beaten eggs and knead the dough. Roll out the dough with a rolling pin. Spray the slow cooker bowl with the olive oil. Place the rolled out dough in the slow cooker.

Sprinkle the dough with the chopped ham and grated Parmesan.

Then sprinkle the pizza with the Italian seasoning. Close the lid and cook the pizza for 3 hours on High.

Then let the cooked pizza cool slightly and serve it!

Nutrition: Calories 320, Fat 24.7, Fiber 3.4, Carbs 8.5, Protein 20.3

5. Breakfast Sweet Pepper Hash

Preparation Time: 15 minutes

Cooking time: 4 hours

Servings: 4

Ingredients:

8 oz ground pork

One onion, chopped

Two sweet peppers, chopped

One teaspoon ghee

¼ cup chicken stock

½ teaspoon chili flakes

4 oz Cheddar cheese

Directions:

Mix the chopped onion and sweet pepper.

Add chickens stock and ghee.

Add the chili flakes and transfer the mix to the slow cooker.

Shred the cheddar cheese and add it to the slow cooker as well.

Add ground pork and stir the ingredients carefully with a spatula.

Close the lid and cook the hash for 4 hours on High.

Stir the meal and serve!

Nutrition: Calories 235, Fat 12.7, Fiber 1.4, Carbs 7.5, Protein 22.8

6. Pork Breakfast Sausages

Preparation Time: 15 minutes

Cooking time: 7 hours

Servings: 3

Ingredients:

9 oz ground pork

1 oz onion, grated

One tablespoon almond flour

One teaspoon coconut flour

¼ teaspoon ground black pepper

¾ teaspoon chili flakes

One teaspoon ghee

Directions:

Mix up together the ground pork and grated onion.

Add almond flour and coconut flour.

Then add ground black pepper and chili flakes.

Stir the mixture well and form small sausages.

Place the sausages in the slow cooker and add the ghee.

Cook the sausages for 7 hours on Low.

When the sausages are cooked, let them cool slightly.

Enjoy!

Nutrition: Calories 188, Fat 9.8, Fiber 2.9, Carbs 5.7, Protein 25.1

7. Potato Breakfast Mix

Preparation time: 10 minutes

Cooking time: 5 hours

Servings: 4

Ingredients:

One tablespoon olive oil

One garlic clove, minced

Two big sweet potatoes, chopped

One yellow onion, chopped

3 cups tomato juice

4 ounces green chilies chopped

2 cups veggie stock

One teaspoon allspice, ground

A pinch of salt and black pepper

Two teaspoons ginger, grated

Directions:

In your slow cooker, mix the oil with the garlic, sweet potatoes, tomato juice, green chilies, stock, allspice, salt, pepper, ginger, toss, cover, and cook on Low for 5 hours.

Stir the mix again, divide between plates and serve for breakfast.

Enjoy!

Nutrition: Calories 203, Fat 3, Fiber 3, Carbs 16, Protein 8

8. Breakfast Veggie Casserole

Preparation time: 10 minutes

Cooking time: 5 hours

Servings: 4

Ingredients:

One yellow onion, chopped

One tablespoon olive oil

Three garlic cloves, minced

One teaspoon smoked paprika

½ teaspoon cumin, ground

Three carrots, sliced

One tablespoon thyme, dried

Two celery stalks, chopped

One red bell pepper, chopped

One yellow bell pepper, chopped

12 ounces canned tomatoes, chopped

5 ounces veggie stock

Two eggplants, chopped

Two thyme sprigs

A pinch of salt and black pepper

Directions:

Grease your slow cooker with the oil, add onion, garlic, paprika, cumin, carrots, thyme, celery, red and yellow bell pepper, tomatoes, stock, thyme, salt, pepper, and top with eggplant slices. Cover, cook on Low for 5 hours, divide between plates and serve for breakfast.

Enjoy!

Nutrition: Calories 200, Fat 2, Fiber 1, carbs 5, protein 10

9. Cheddar Jalapeno Breakfast Sausages

Preparation time: 5 minutes

Cooking time: 6 hours

Servings: 12

Ingredients:

12 medium-sized breakfast sausages

One jalapeno pepper, chopped

½ cup cheddar cheese, grated

¼ cup heavy cream

Salt and pepper to taste

Directions:

Mix all items in a bowl, then put it into the slow cooker.

Set to cook on Low for 6 hours or on high for 4 hours.

Garnish with parsley on top.

Nutrition: Calories: 472 Carbohydrates: 1.2 Protein: 32.6 Fat: 42.4 Sugar: 0 Fiber: 0.4

10. Breakfast Veggie Salad

Preparation time: 10 minutes

Cooking time: 5 hours

Servings: 4

Ingredients:

Six tomatoes halved

Two red onions cut into quarters

Four long red peppers, cut into strips

Two yellow peppers, cut into wedges

Six garlic cloves

One tablespoon baby capers, drained

One teaspoon sweet paprika

A pinch of salt and black pepper

Four tablespoons olive oil

Juice of ½ lemon

Directions:

Add the oil to your slow cooker, add tomatoes, onions, long peppers, yellow peppers, garlic, capers, paprika, salt, pepper, lemon juice, toss, cover, and cook low for 5 hours.

Divide into bowls and serve for breakfast.

Enjoy!

Nutrition: Calories 189, Fat 3, Fiber 4, Carbs 14, Protein 7

11. Breakfast Pork and Avocado Mix

Preparation time: 10 minutes

Cooking time: 10 hours

Servings: 4

Ingredients:

4 pounds pork butt roast

One tablespoon cumin powder

Two tablespoons chili powder

One teaspoon coriander, ground

One tablespoon oregano, dried

Two yellow onions, sliced

Two avocados, peeled, pitted, and sliced

Directions:

In your slow cooker, mix pork butt with chili, cumin, oregano, coriander, and onions, toss, cover, and cook on Low for 10 hours. Shred meat, divide between plates, top with avocado slices, and serve for breakfast.

Enjoy!

Nutrition: Calories 270, Fat 4, Fiber 10, Carbs 8, Protein 25

CHAPTER 8:

Lunch Recipes

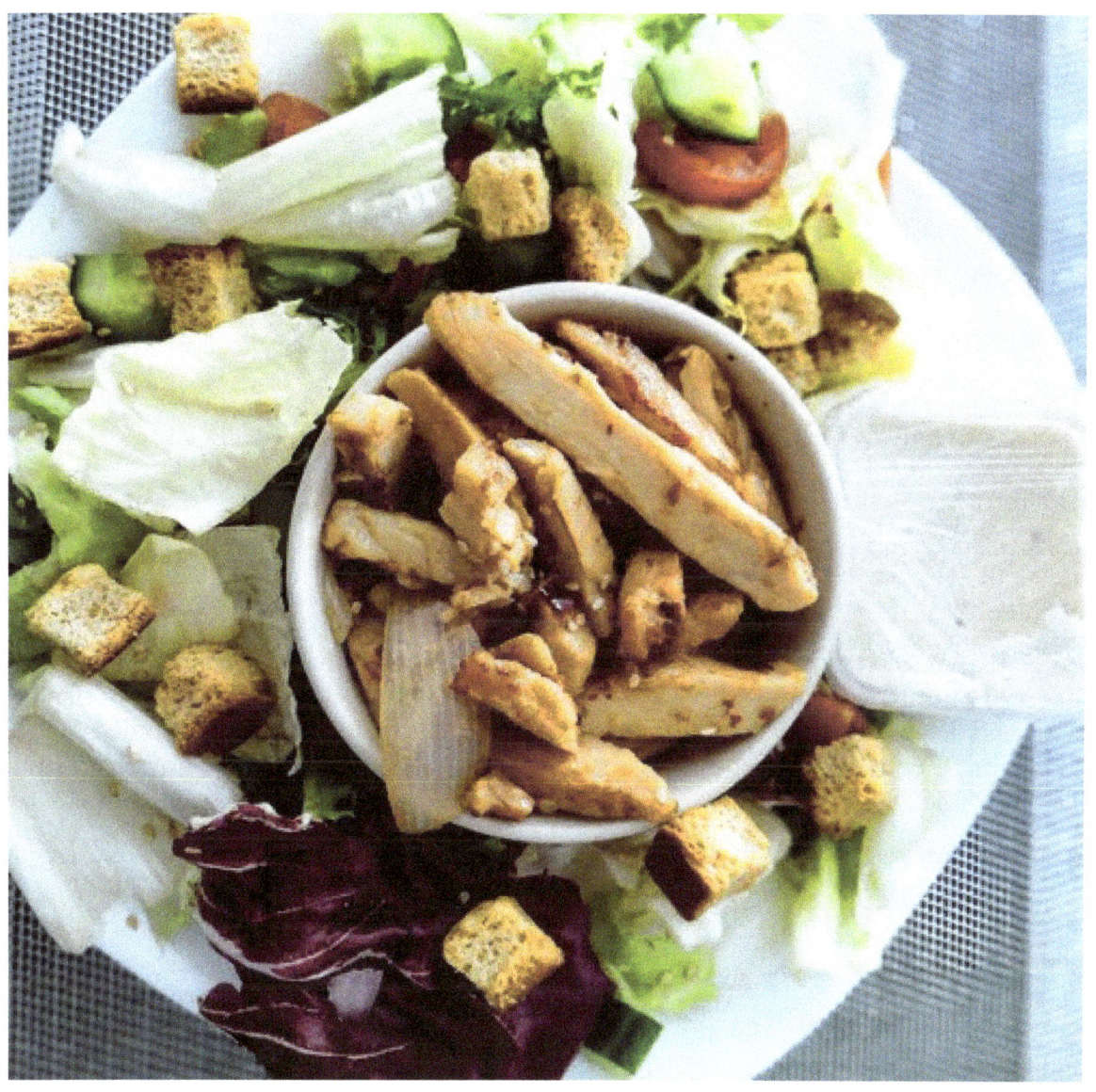

12. Lime Chicken with Savoy Cabbage

Preparation time: 10 minutes

Cooking time: 7 hours

Servings: 4

Ingredients:

Eight chicken thighs, skinless

2 cups Savoy cabbage, chopped

One stalk celery, diced

One medium onion, diced

1 tbsp ginger, grated

½ cup chicken stock

Two limes

1 tsp salt

1 tsp black pepper

Extra virgin olive oil

Spicy squash noodles for serving

Directions:

Place 4 tbsp extra virgin olive oil in a slow cooker, spread around the bottom. Add the ginger and onions. Slice lime into ½" thick circles. Place chicken in the bottom of a slow cooker, and sprinkle with ½ tsp salt and ½ tsp black pepper. Top with lime slices. On top of those, place celery and cabbage. Pour in chicken stock, and cook on Low for 7 hours. Serve with Spicy Squash Noodles.

Nutrition: Calories 273 Carbs 5.7 g Fat 12 g Protein 34 g Sodium 689 mg Sugar 0 g

13. Middle Eastern Lamb Zucchini Casserole

Preparation time: 20 minutes

Cooking time: 7 hours

Servings: 6

Ingredients:

4 zucchinis, peeled

1 lb ground lamb

½ cup coconut cream

2 eggs

¼ cup Parmesan

½ tsp cinnamon

½ tsp cloves

½ tsp cumin

1 tsp salt

1 tsp black pepper

Extra virgin olive oil

Directions:

Use a mandolin, thinly-slice zucchini lengthwise. Heat 3 tbsp extra virgin olive oil in the skillet. Add lamb, cinnamon, cloves, and cumin. Brown. Combine coconut cream with egg, salt, and black pepper. Coat slow cooker with olive oil, place ¼ of zucchini strips on the slow cooker's bottom. Next, brush coconut cream mixture on zucchini. Place another layer of zucchini and half the remaining coconut cream, top with lamb, another layer of zucchini, remaining coconut cream. Cook on Low for 7 hours.

Nutrition: Calories 203 Carbs 4.7 g Fat 10 g Protein 25 g Sodium 479 mg Sugar 0 g

14. Ginger Steak Broccoli

Preparation time: 10 minutes

Cooking time: 4 hours

Servings: 4

Ingredients:

1 lb sirloin steak

3 cups broccoli florets (frozen okay)

1 cup low-sodium beef stock

1 tbsp grated ginger

½ tsp thyme

1 tsp salt

1 tsp black pepper

Extra virgin olive oil

Directions:

Slice sirloin steak against the grain into ½" wide strips.

Place 4 tbsp extra virgin olive oil in a skillet, add steak, and brown for a minute on each side.

Place steak, broccoli florets, along with ginger, beef stock, and soy sauce in a slow cooker.

Cook on medium-high for 4 hours.

Enjoy alone or with cauliflower rice.

Nutrition: Calories 273 Carbs 6 g Fat 11 g Protein 37 g Sodium 714 mg Sugar 0 g

15. BLT Chicken Salad

Preparation time: 20 minutes

Cooking time: 4 hours

Servings: 4

Ingredients:

4 x 4oz chicken breast

2 cup low-sodium chicken broth

Eight slices bacon

2 cups romaine lettuce

One tomato, diced

1 tsp salt

1 tsp black pepper

¼ cup organic mayonnaise

Extra virgin olive oil

Directions:

Coat slow cooker with a little olive oil, and set on high.

Tenderize chicken breast, and sprinkle each chicken breast with salt and black pepper.

Wrap each chicken breast with bacon, and place it in a slow cooker.

Cook chicken breast on high for 4 hours.

Place mayonnaise with 1 tsp black pepper and 4 tbsp extra virgin olive oil in a blender. Mix until smooth.

Combine lettuce, tomato in a bowl, and toss with mayo dressing.

Top salad with chicken breast and serve.

Nutrition: Calories 366 Carbs 6 g Fat 19 g Protein 43 g Sodium 1183 mg Sugar 0 g

16.   Figs and Goat Cheese-Stuffed Chicken

Preparation time: 20 minutes

Cooking time: 8 hours

Servings: 4

Ingredients:

4 x 4oz chicken breasts

4 figs

½ cup goat cheese, crumbled

1 tsp salt

1 tsp black pepper

Extra virgin olive oil

Directions:

Combine 3 tbsp olive oil, salt, black pepper in a bowl, and rub onto chicken breasts. Marinate for an hour.

Remove fig skin, and slice figs into ½" pieces. Combine with goat cheese.

Turn slow cooker to Low.

Place plastic wrap over chicken breasts and pound with a mallet until each breast is approximately ¼" thick (or ask your butcher to do it).

Scoop a quarter of the cheese-fig mixture into the chicken, roll up chicken breast, and place in a slow cooker.

Repeat for each chicken breast.

Cook on low for 8 hours.

Serve with a green salad.

Nutrition: Calories 369 Carbs 7 g Fat 18 g Protein 46 g Sodium 811 mg Sugar 0 g

17. Carne Asada

Preparation Time: 10 minutes

Cooking Time: 8 hours

Servings: 8

Ingredients:

4 lb chuck roast

1 onion, chopped

4 limes, juiced

½ cup cilantro, minced

8 cloves garlic, minced

2 tsp paprika

2 tsp oregano

2 tsp cumin

2 tsp salt

1 tsp black pepper

Directions:

Rinse pot roast and pat dry.

Combine remaining ingredients in a blender, and mix until well combined.

Brush slow cooker with extra virgin olive oil, and set on high.

Coat pot roast with cilantro topping.

Place in a slow cooker, and cook for 8 hours.

Serve with Cauliflower Rice.

Nutrition: Calories 506 Carbs 3 g Fat 19 g Protein 75 g Sodium 733 mg Sugar 0 g

18. Amazing Pulled Pork

Preparation Time: 25 minutes

Cooking Time: 8 hours

Servings: 8

Ingredients:

5 lb pork shoulder

2 tbsp mustard

2 cups tomato purée

6 Medjool Dates, pitted

½ tsp cloves, ground

½ tsp cinnamon

2 tsp salt

Extra virgin olive oil

Tortilla Wraps

Eight eggs

1 tbsp coconut flour

½ tsp salt

Directions:

Place pitted dates in a blender, mix until paste forms, add tomato purée, cinnamon, salt, black pepper, and mix. Combine mustard, blended tomato puree, cloves, cinnamon, salt, and mix.

Place pork shoulder in a slow cooker, pour the sauce into a slow cooker, and coat pork shoulder. Cook pork for 8 hours on high.

Once the pork is cooked, use a fork to shred.

For tortilla wraps, whisk eggs, add milk and flour, and mix until well combined.

Heat 4 tbsp oil in a skillet on medium-high.

Pour 1/8th of the mixture into skillet and cook each side 30 seconds.

Spoon pork mixture into egg tortilla and serve.

Nutrition: Calories 777 Carbs 8 g Fat 55 g Protein 59 g Sodium 835 mg Sugar 5 g

19. Braised Pork Belly

Preparation Time: 10 minutes

Cooking Time: 4 hours

Servings: 8

Ingredients:

1 lb pork belly

Two medium onions, diced

1 tsp Dijon mustard

½ cup apple sauce

1 tsp black pepper

1 tsp salt

Directions:

Heat extra virgin olive oil in the skillet, add onion, sauté for a minute.

Place onion in a slow cooker, add pork belly, apple sauce—cook on high for 4 hours.

Serve with Walnut Cabbage Salad.

Nutrition: Calories 278 Carbs 3.5 g Fat 15 g Protein 26 g Sodium 1214 mg Sugar 0 g

20. Peppercorn Short Ribs

Preparation Time: 10 minutes

Cooking Time: 4 hours

Servings: 8

Ingredients:

4 lbs short ribs, bone-in

Eight peppercorns

2 cups low-sodium beef

One onion, diced

Two carrots, peeled, diced

Two celery stalks, diced

Four cloves, minced

1 tsp thyme

1 tsp rosemary

Two bay leaves

2 tsp salt

2 tsp black pepper

Extra virgin olive oil

Directions:

Heat 4 tbsp extra virgin olive oil in a skillet. Add onions and garlic, and sauté until brown.

Place onion mixture in a slow cooker, add short ribs, carrots, celery stalk, cloves, thyme, rosemary, peppercorns, bay leaves, salt, and black pepper.

Cook on high for 4 hours.

Nutrition: Calories 520 Carbs 3.7 g Fat 24 g Protein 67 g Sodium 923 mg Sugar 0 g

[Handwritten note: make ½ recipe, use ½ the amount of spicy sausage]

21. Spicy Italian Sausage and Zucchini Noodles

Preparation Time: 20 minutes

Cooking Time: 4 hours

Servings: 6

Ingredients:

6 Spicy Italian pork sausages

One onion, peeled and diced

2 cups low-sodium chicken stock

One tomato, diced

Four zucchinis, peeled

1 tsp oregano

1 tsp salt

1 tsp black pepper

Extra virgin olive oil

Directions:

Coat slow cooker with a little extra virgin olive oil, and set to high.

Slice sausage into ½" thick rounds, and place in a slow cooker. Heat 3 tbsp extra virgin olive oil in a skillet, add onion and garlic, sauté for a minute, and add to slow cooker. Add tomatoes, oregano, and a tsp of salt and black pepper along with the chicken stock, cover, and cook for 4 hours. Using Mandolin, slice zucchini vertically to create thin Zucchini Noodles. Top zucchini noodles with Spicy Italian Sausage and serve.

Nutrition: Calories 254 Carbs 8.5 g Fat 14 g Protein 24 g Sodium 1044 mg Sugar 3 g

22. Meaty Cauliflower Lasagna

Preparation Time: 20 minutes

Cooking Time: 5 hours

Servings: 8

Ingredients:

1 lb ground beef

One small cauliflower head

One red onion, diced

Four cloves garlic, minced

2 cups crushed tomato

1 cup Mozzarella, shredded

One egg

1 tsp oregano

One bay leaf

1 tsp black pepper

1 tsp salt

Extra virgin olive oil

Directions:

Brush slow cooker with olive oil, and set the slow cooker on medium-high.

Separate cauliflower into florets, peel the outer layer of cauliflower stem and dice stem.

Place cauliflower in the food processor, pulse into rice-like granules, crack an egg into cauliflower, and mix along with ½ tsp of salt.

Place 3 tbsp olive oil in a skillet, add ground beef, brown, add crushed tomatoes, oregano, bay leaf, black pepper, and ½ tsp salt, mix.

Place ½ cauliflower mixture in a slow cooker, next layer ⅓ of beef mixture and ½ of cheese, place remaining cauliflower on top. Spoon remaining sauce on top of the cauliflower, sprinkle with remaining cheese. Cook on medium-high for 5 hours.

Nutrition: Calories 342 Carbs 8.2 g Fat 14 g Protein 45 g Sodium 681 mg Sugar 0 g

23. Chili Verde

Preparation Time: 10 minutes

Cooking Time: 7 hours

Servings: 8

Ingredients:

1½ lbs pork shoulder

½ lb sirloin, cubed

4 Anaheim chiles, stemmed

Six cloves garlic, minced

½ cup cilantro, chopped

Two onions, peeled and sliced

Two tomatoes, chopped.

1 tbsp tomato paste

One lime

1 tbsp cumin

1 tbsp oregano

Extra virgin olive oil

Directions:

Slice pork shoulder into ½" cubes, and set slow cooker to medium. Heat 4 tbsp extra virgin olive oil in a skillet, add onions, Anaheim chilies, garlic, and sauté for 2 minutes.

Place skillet mixture into a slow cooker, add pork shoulder, sirloin, and stir.

Add tomatoes, cilantro, tomato paste, cumin, oregano, and salt to the pot.

Cover and cook for 7 hours.

Squeeze a little lime in each bowl when serving.

Nutrition: Calories 262 Carbs 6 g Fat 16 g Protein 23 g Sodium 63 mg Sugar 0 g

24. Tandoori Salmon with Fresh Cucumber Salad

Preparation Time: 10 minutes

Cooking Time: 3 hours

Servings: 8

Ingredients:

4 x 4oz Wild salmon fillets

2 tsp Tandoori spice

1 tsp salt

1 tsp black pepper

4 tbsp ghee

Cucumber Salad

1 English cucumber

1 cup arugula

½ cup parsley

¼ cup lemon juice

2 tbsp extra virgin olive oil

Directions:

Heat ghee in a skillet over medium heat along with tandoori spice for a minute.

Place salmon fillets in a slow cooker, skin side down, sprinkle with salt, black pepper, and pour Tandoori butter over salmon.

Cook on high for 3.5 hours.

Meanwhile, salmon cook, dice the cucumber and toss with arugula, parsley, lemon juice, and extra virgin olive oil.

Serve salmon with fresh cucumber salad.

Nutrition: Calories 413 Carbs 4 g Fat 34 g Protein 25 g Sodium 645 mg Sugar 0 g

CHAPTER 9:

Snack Recipes

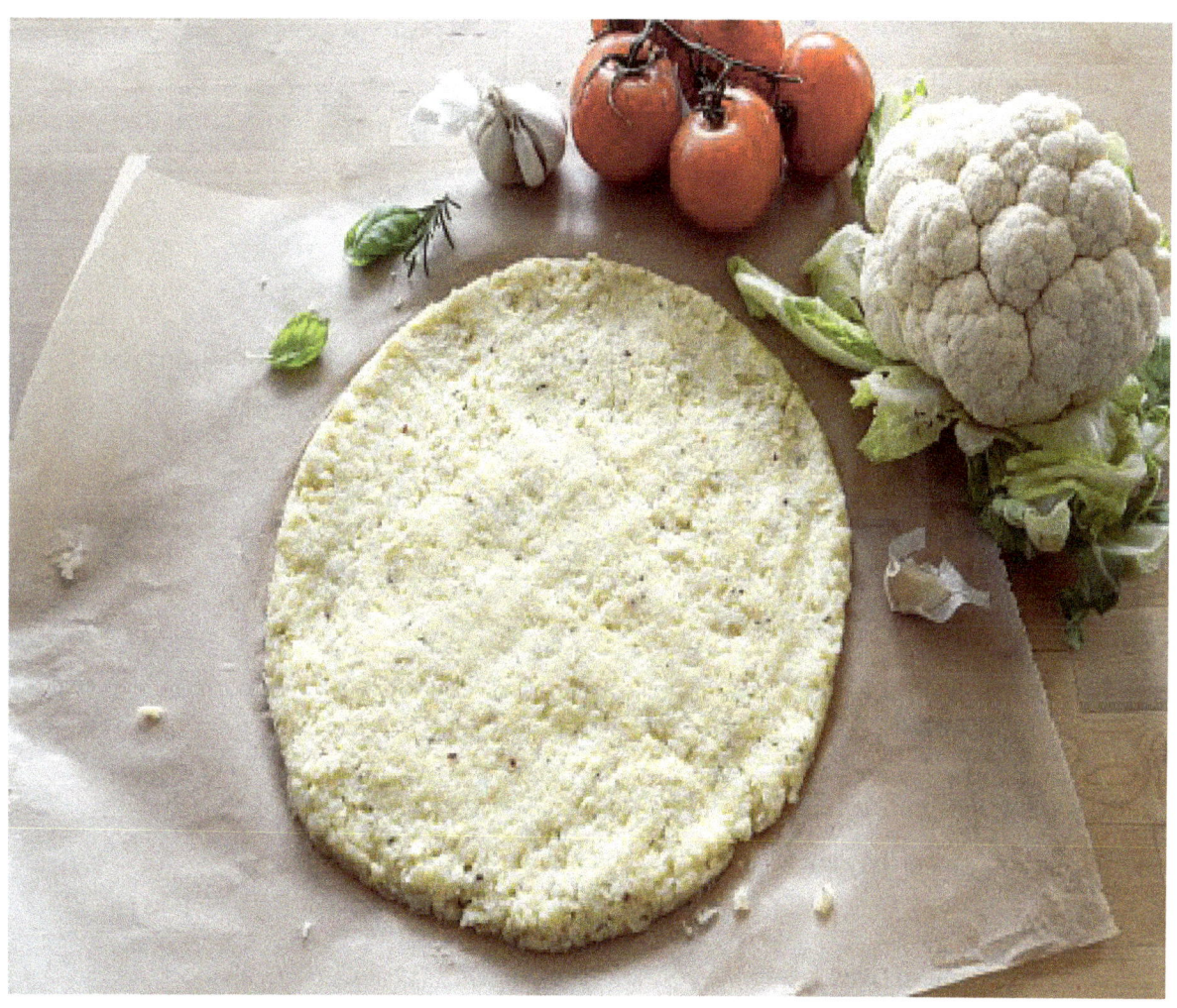

25. Chicken Bites

Preparation time: 15 minutes

Cooking time: 4 hours

Servings: 4

Ingredients:

1-pound chicken fillet, roughly cubed

One teaspoon turmeric powder

One teaspoon yellow curry paste

1 oz Parmesan, grated

¼ cup butter

Directions:

In the slow cooker, mix the chicken with the curry paste and the other ingredients and toss. Close the lid and the chicken tenders for 4 hours on High.

Nutrition: Carbs 3.5, Protein 16.5

Calories 336, Fat 13.7, Fiber 2.6,

26. Paprika Almonds

Preparation time: 10 minutes

Cooking time: 6 hours

Servings: 2

Ingredients: 1 cup almonds

One tablespoon sweet paprika

1/3 cup water

½ teaspoon Vanilla extract

¾ teaspoon ground ginger

Directions:

In the slow cooker, mix the almonds with the other ingredients, toss and close the lid.

Cook the almonds for 6 hours on Low. Mix up the almonds every 1 hour.

Nutrition: Calories 126, Fat 4.3, Fiber 2.1, Carbs 9.1, Protein 5.2

27. Mixed Nuts

Preparation time: 15 minutes

Cooking time: 3 hours

Servings: 6

Ingredients:

1 cup almonds

1 cup walnuts

1 cup sunflower seeds

1/4 cup water

Two tablespoons poppy seeds

One teaspoon sweet paprika

One teaspoon lemon zest, grated

Directions:

In the slow cooker, mix the almonds with walnuts and the other ingredients, toss and close the lid.

Cook for 3 hours on High.

Divide into bowls and serve.

Nutrition: Calories 137, Fat 7.9, Fiber 2.3, Carbs 5.1, Protein 7.2

28. Beef and Zucchini Wraps

Preparation time: 15 minutes

Cooking time: 4 hours

Servings: 6

Ingredients:

Six keto tortillas

Two zucchinis, roughly cubed

1-pound beef sirloin, chopped

One teaspoon sweet paprika

Five tablespoons cream cheese

One teaspoon butter

One teaspoon garam masala

Directions:

In the slow cooker, mix the zucchinis with the other ingredients except for the tortillas, stir and close the slow cooker lid. Cook beef for 4 hours on High. Divide this on each tortilla, wrap and serve.

Nutrition: Calories 278, Fat 8.3, Fiber 4.3, Carbs 8.8, Protein 23.7

29. Cauliflower Bites

Preparation time: 10 minutes

Cooking time: 3 hours

Servings: 5

Ingredients:

2 cups cauliflower florets

¾ cup coconut cream

4 oz Parmesan, grated

One teaspoon turmeric powder

One teaspoon paprika

One teaspoon butter, melted

Directions:

In the slow cooker, mix the cauliflower with the cream and the other ingredients and close it. Cook the cauliflower bites for 3 hours on High.

Nutrition: Calories 202, Fat 6.6, Fiber 5,.4, Carbs 2.9, Protein 9.2

30. Mushroom Skewers

Preparation time: 15 minutes

Cooking time: 4 hours

Servings: 4

Ingredients:

6 oz white mushrooms, roughly chopped

1 eggplant, peeled

1 tablespoon butter, melted

1 teaspoon minced garlic

1 teaspoon dried parsley

½ teaspoon ground black pepper

Directions:

Chop the eggplant roughly. Mix the white mushrooms, eggplant, minced garlic, dried parsley, and ground black pepper. Stir the vegetables and slide them onto skewers. Place the skewers in the slow cooker and add butter. Cook the skewers for 4 hours on Low. Serve the meal!

Nutrition: Calories 65, Fat 3.2, Fiber 4.6, Carbs 8.6, Protein 2.6

31. Cheese Sticks

Preparation time: 20 minutes

Cooking time: 2.5 hours

Servings: 8

Ingredients:

Four eggs, beaten

1 cup Cheddar cheese, shredded

One tablespoon fresh dill, chopped

One tablespoon chives, chopped

One teaspoon turmeric powder

One teaspoon butter softened

1/3 cup almond flour

One teaspoon salt

Directions:

In the mixing bowl, mix up together beaten eggs, cheese, and the other ingredients. You should get a soft homogenous mixture.

Line the bottom of the slow cooker with the baking paper.

Transfer the cheese mixture to the slow cooker and flatten well.

Close the lid and bake it for 2.5 hours on High.

Then chill the cooked mixture very well and cut into the serving sticks.

Nutrition: Calories 304, Fat 8.3, Fiber 4.5, Carbs 1.6, Protein 7

32. Eggplant Bread

Preparation time: 15 minutes

Cooking time: 7 hours

Servings: 4

Ingredients:

Two eggplants, chopped

Two eggs, beaten

Three tablespoons coconut cream

One teaspoon garam masala

Two tablespoons almond flour

½ teaspoon baking soda

One teaspoon lime juice

½ teaspoon ground black pepper

One teaspoon butter, melted

Directions:

Line the slow cooker bottom with the baking paper.

In the mixing bowl, mix up together eggs with the eggplants and the other ingredients, and stir well.

Transfer the eggplant bread mixture to the slow cooker and flatten it well.

Close the lid and cook zucchini bread for 7 hours on Low.

Nutrition: Calories 186, Fat 12.1, Fiber 4.6, Carbs 11.2, Protein 7.5

33. Almond Granola

Preparation time: 10 minutes

Cooking time: 1.5 hour

Servings: 6

Ingredients:

1/3 cup coconut shred

1/4 cup almonds, chopped

Two eggs whisked

One tablespoon almond flour

One teaspoon Erythritol

One teaspoon ground cinnamon

Directions:

In the slow cooker, mix the almonds with the coconut and the other ingredients, stir and spread into the pot. Cook granola on High for 1 hour. Then mix up the granola mixture well and cook it for 30 minutes more. Chill the cooked granola well and store it in the glass jar.

Nutrition: Calories 203, Fat 12.3, Fiber 3.1, Carbs 5.9, Protein 4.7

34. Chili Walnuts

Preparation time: 10 minutes

Cooking time: 2 hours

Servings: 3

Ingredients:

1 cup walnuts

One teaspoon hot paprika

One teaspoon salt

One egg white

½ teaspoon chili powder

Directions:

Whisk the egg white, paprika, salt, and chili until you get foam.

Coat walnuts in the egg white mixture.

Line the slow cooker bottom with baking paper and arrange coated walnuts.

Cook them for 2 hours on High.

Nutrition: Calories 270, Fat 10.1, Fiber 4.7, Carbs 6.3, Protein 5.8

35. Pork Bites

Preparation time: 15 minutes

Cooking time: 4 hours

Servings: 4

Ingredients:

1 cup pork stew meat, cubed

One teaspoon keto tomato sauce

One teaspoon chili flakes

¼ cup heavy cream

One teaspoon olive oil

½ teaspoon salt

Directions:

In the slow cooker, mix the pork cubes with tomato paste and the other ingredients, close the lid and cook for 4 hours on High.

Divide into bowls and serve

Nutrition: Calories 283, Fat 20.2, Fiber 3.3, Carbs 1.4, Protein 14.5

36. Turkey Meatballs

Preparation time: 15 minutes

Cooking time: 4 hours

Servings: 3

Ingredients:

½ cup ground turkey meat

One egg whisked

One teaspoon oregano, dried

One teaspoon curry powder

½ teaspoon ground black pepper

¼ teaspoon salt

¾ cup of coconut milk

Directions:

In the mixing bowl, mix up the meat with the egg and the other ingredients except for the coconut milk. Stir and shape small meatballs out of this mix.

Pour the coconut milk into the slow cooker, add the meatballs and toss gently.

Cook the meatballs for 4 hours on High.

Nutrition: Calories 273, Fat 16.7, Fiber 1.5, Carbs 4.1, Protein 11.8

37. Tomato Salmon Meatballs

Preparation time: 15 minutes

Cooking time: 3 hours

Servings: 2

Ingredients:

6 oz salmon fillet, minced

One tablespoon keto tomato sauce

One teaspoon almond flour

½ teaspoon turmeric

¾ teaspoon salt

¼ teaspoon sweet paprika

¼ cup organic almond milk

One teaspoon butter

Directions:

In a bowl, mix the salmon meat with the keto tomato sauce and the other ingredients except for the milk and butter, stir and make small meatballs.

Place them in the slow cooker, add butter and almond milk. Close the lid of the slow cooker.

Cook the appetizer for 3 hours on High.

Nutrition: Calories 301, Fat 9.7, Fiber 2.7, Carbs 5.4, Protein 15.8

38. Pecans Bowls

Preparation time: 7 minutes

Cooking time: 1 hour

Servings: 6

Ingredients:

Six pecans

One teaspoon butter, melted

One tablespoon keto tomato sauce

½ teaspoon olive oil

Directions:

In the slow cooker, mix the pecans with the keto tomato sauce and the other ingredients, toss and close the lid.

Cook pecans for 1 hour on High. Stir the pecans after 30 minutes of cooking and divide them into bowls at the end.

Nutrition: Calories 126, Fat 11.2, Fiber 1.5, Carbs 2, Protein 1.5

39. Sausage Dip

Preparation time: 10 minutes

Cooking time: 4 hours

Servings: 5

Ingredients:

1 cup Italian sausages, crumbled

One tablespoon chives, chopped

One teaspoon Italian seasoning

One teaspoon sweet paprika

1 cup Cheddar cheese, shredded

1 cup Mozzarella cheese, shredded

¼ cup heavy cream

Directions:

In the slow cooker, mix the sausages with chives and the other ingredients and stir.

Close the lid and cook dip for 4 hours on Low.

Nutrition: Calories 304, Fat 24.9, Fiber 5.4, Carbs 6.5, Protein 13.8

40. Butter Pork Ribs

Preparation time: 15 minutes

Cooking time: 7 hours

Servings: 4

Ingredients:

10 oz pork ribs

Three tablespoons butter, soft

1/3 cup coconut cream

One teaspoon turmeric powder

½ teaspoon salt

One teaspoon garlic powder

Directions:

In the slow cooker, mix the pork with soft butter and the other ingredients.

Close the lid and cook the pork ribs for 7 hours on Low.

Nutrition: Calories 321, Fat 14.8, Fiber 4.5, Carbs 6.5, Protein 19.7

41. Chicken Dip

Preparation time: 15 minutes

Cooking time: 4 hours

Servings: 4

Ingredients:

1 cup ground chicken

One teaspoon chives, chopped

½ cup keto tomato sauce

One tablespoon olive oil

One teaspoon basil, dried

¼ teaspoon minced garlic

3 oz Parmesan, grated

Directions:

In the slow cooker, mix the chicken with the tomato sauce and the other ingredients, whisk and close the lid.

Cook the dip for 4 hours on High, divide into bowls and serve.

Nutrition: Calories 236, Fat 7.2, Fiber 5.1, Carbs 6.5, Protein 17

CHAPTER 10:

Dinner Recipes

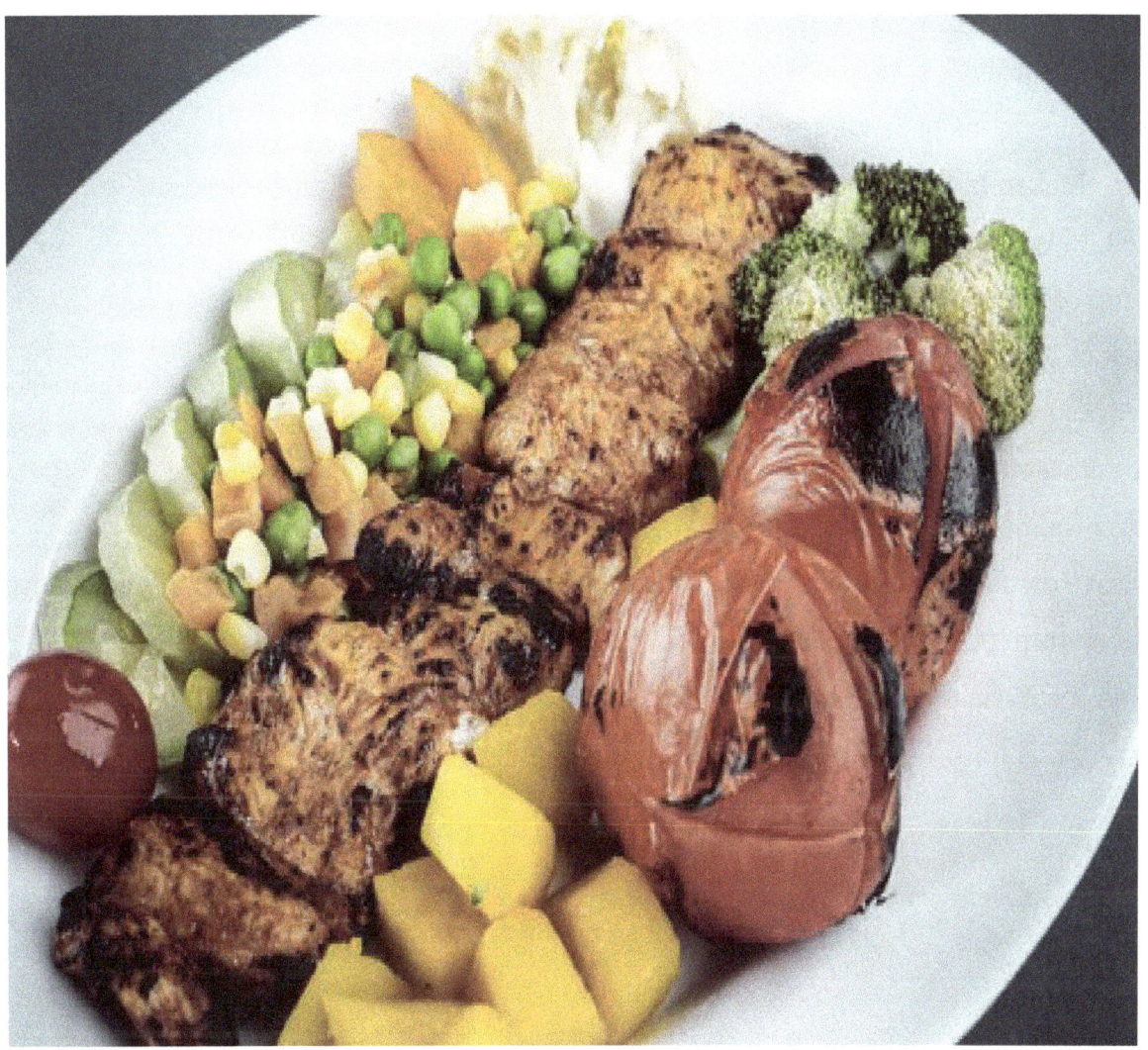

42. Paprika Pork Tenderloin

Preparation time: 15 minutes

Cooking time: 4 hours & 20 minutes

Servings: 4

Ingredients:

1 ½ lb. lean pork tenderloin

½ teaspoon salt

Two tablespoons paprika, smoked

1 cup chicken broth

One tablespoon oregano

½ cup of salsa

Black pepper

Directions:

Pour chicken stock into a small mixing bowl.

Add salsa, pepper, paprika, salt, and oregano. Mix well.

Remove the fat from the pork before placing it in the slow cooker. Add the liquid mixture.

Cook within 4 hours on high.

Shred the pork, then cook for another 20 minutes without cover.

Nutrition: Calories: 160 Carbs: 2g Fat: 8g Protein: 22g

43. Pork Carnitas

Preparation time: 15 minutes

Cooking time: 8 hours

Servings: 16

Ingredients:

8 lb. Boston pork butt

1 cup of water

Two tablespoons butter

Two tablespoons chili powder

Four tablespoons garlic, minced

One large onion, sliced thin

One tablespoon pepper

Two tablespoons cumin

One tablespoon salt

Two tablespoons thyme

Directions:

Grease the slow cooker using butter. Distribute onion and garlic evenly in the bottom of the slow cooker.

Remove the fat from the meat and lightly slice the top with a crisscross pattern. Mix the spices in a bowl, then coat the meat with it.

Put meat in the slow cooker with water—Cook for about 8 hours, high.

Nutrition: Calories: 200 Carbs: 0g Fat: 14g Protein: 20g

Lemongrass Coconut Pulled Pork

Preparation Time: 15 minutes

Cooking Time: 8 hours

- 3 lb. butt roast or pork loin
- ½ cup of coconut milk
- 2-inch ginger, sliced
- Three tablespoons lemongrass, minced
- One onion, sliced
- Three cloves garlic, minced
- One teaspoon ground pepper
- Two teaspoons kosher salt
- One tablespoon apple cider vinegar
- Three tablespoons olive oil

Directions:

Remove fat from the roast and cut a crisscross pattern into it. Distribute onion and ginger slices evenly at the bottom of a slow cooker.

Mix olive oil, pepper, salt, apple cider vinegar, lemongrass, and garlic in a bowl until a loose paste is formed. Coat the pork with the mixture and put it in the slow cooker.

Cover and leave it overnight. Once done, pour coconut milk into the slow cooker and set it on low—Cook for 8 hours. Shred the meat using forks.

Nutrition: Calories: 120 Carbs: 0g Fat: 3g Protein: 23g

45. Cheesy Cauliflower Gratin

Preparation time: 15 minutes

Cooking time: 4 hours & 10 minutes

Servings: 3

Ingredients:

2 cups cauliflower florets

Three tablespoons heavy whipping cream

Three deli slices pepper Jack cheese

Two tablespoons butter

Salt to taste

Pepper to taste

Directions:

Add cauliflower, cream, butter, salt, and pepper into the slow cooker. Close the lid. Cook on 'Low' for 3-4 hours or until tender.

When done, mash with a fork. Taste and adjust the seasoning if necessary.

Place cheese slices on top. Cover and cook within 10 minutes or until cheese melts. Serve right away.

Nutrition: Calories 216 Fat 19.3g Carbohydrate 4g Protein 5.7g

46. Creamy Ricotta Spaghetti Squash

Preparation time: 15 minutes

Cooking time: 6 hours

Servings: 8

Ingredients:

Two spaghetti squash, halved, deseeded

Two teaspoons garlic powder

Four tablespoons fresh basil or parsley, chopped

2 cups part-skim ricotta cheese

Two teaspoons lemon zest, grated

Salt to taste

Pepper to taste

Cooking spray

Directions:

Spray the cut part of the spaghetti squash with cooking spray. Place it in the slow cooker with the cut side facing down.

Close the lid. Cook on 'Low' for 4-6 hours or until tender. When done, using a fork, scrape the squash, and add into a bowl.

Add ricotta cheese, lemon zest, garlic powder, salt, pepper, and basil and mix well.

Nutrition: Calories112 Fat 5.4g Carbohydrate 9.1g Protein 7.7g

47. Creamy Keto Mash

Preparation time: 15 minutes

Cooking time: 2 hours

Servings: 8

Ingredients:

Two large heads of cauliflower, chopped into small floret's

Four cloves garlic, minced

One large onion, chopped

Eight tablespoons butter or ghee+ extra to top

1 cup cream cheese or sour cream

½ cup of water

Salt to taste

Pepper to taste

Directions:

Place the cauliflower florets in the slow cooker. Pour about ½ a cup of water.

Close the lid. Cook on 'Low' for 1-2 hours or until tender.

Place a skillet over medium heat. Add two tablespoons of butter or ghee. When it melts, add onions and garlic and sauté until the onions are translucent.

Add remaining butter and stir, then remove from heat. Transfer into a blender. Add cauliflower and blend until smooth or blend in the food processor. Add cream cheese and pulse until well combined. Transfer into a bowl, then add salt and pepper to taste. Top with butter plus ghee and serve.

Nutrition: Calories 219 Fat 21.7g Carbohydrate 4.3g Protein 3.1g

48. Moist and Spicy Pulled Chicken Breast

Preparation time: 15 minutes

Cooking time: 6 hours

Servings: 8

Ingredients:

One teaspoon dry oregano

One teaspoon dry thyme

One teaspoon dried rosemary

One teaspoon garlic powder

One teaspoon sweet paprika

½ teaspoon chili powder

Salt and pepper to taste

Four tablespoons butter

5.5 pounds of chicken breasts

1 ½ cups ready-made tomato salsa

2 Tablespoons of olive oil

Directions:

Mix dry seasoning, sprinkle half on the bottom of crockpot.

Place the chicken breasts over it, sprinkle the rest of the spices.

Pour the salsa over the chicken. Cover, cook on low for 6 hours.

Nutrition: Calories: 42 Carbs: 1g Fat: 1g Protein: 9g

49. Whole Roasted Chicken

Preparation time: 15 minutes

Cooking time: 8 hours

Servings: 6

Ingredients:

One whole chicken (approximately 5.5 pounds)

Four garlic cloves

Six small onions

1 Tablespoon olive oil, for rubbing

Two teaspoons salt

Two teaspoons sweet paprika

One teaspoon Cayenne pepper

One teaspoon onion powder

One teaspoon ground thyme

Two teaspoons fresh ground black pepper

4 Tablespoons butter, cut into cubes

Directions:

Mix all dry ingredients well.

Stuff the chicken belly with garlic and onions.

On the bottom of the crockpot, place four balls of aluminum foil.

Set the chicken on top of the balls. Rub it generously with olive oil.

Cover the chicken with seasoning, drop in butter pieces. Cover, cook on low for 8 hours.

Nutrition: Calories: 120 Carbs: 1g Fat: 6g Protein: 17g

50. Pot Roast Beef Brisket

Preparation time: 15 minutes

Cooking time: 12 hours

Servings: 10

Ingredients:

6.6 pounds beef brisket, whole

2 Tablespoons olive oil

2 Tablespoons apple cider vinegar

One teaspoon dry oregano

One teaspoon dry thyme

One teaspoon dried rosemary

2 Tablespoons paprika

One teaspoon Cayenne pepper

One tablespoon salt

One teaspoon fresh ground black pepper

Directions:

In a bowl, mix dry seasoning, add olive oil, apple cider vinegar.

Place the meat in the crockpot, generously coat with seasoning mix.

Cover, cook on low for 12 hours.

Remove the brisket, place it on a pan. Sear it under the broiler for 2-4 minutes, observe it so the meat doesn't burn.

Wrap it using a foil, then let it rest for 1 hour. Slice and serve.

Nutrition: Calories: 280 Carbs: 4g Fat: 20g Protein: 20g

51. Seriously Delicious Lamb Roast

Preparation time: 15 minutes

Cooking time: 8 hours

Servings: 8

Ingredients:

12 medium radishes, scrubbed, washed, and cut in half

Salt and pepper to taste

One red onion, diced

Two garlic cloves, minced

One lamb joint (approximately 4.5 pounds) at room temperature

2 Tablespoons olive oil

One teaspoon dry oregano

One teaspoon dry thyme

One sprig of fresh rosemary

4 cups heated broth, your choice

Directions:

Place cut radishes along the bottom of the crockpot. Season. Add onion and garlic.

Blend the herbs plus olive oil in a small bowl until it forms to paste.

Place the meat on top of the radishes. Knead the paste over the meat.

Heat the stock, pour it around the meat.

Cover, cook on low for 8 hours. Let it rest for 20 minutes. Slice and serve.

Nutrition: Calories: 206 Carbs: 4g Fat: 9g Protein: 32g

52. Lamb Provençal

Preparation time: 15 minutes

Cooking time: 8 hours

Servings: 4

Ingredients:

Two racks lamb, approximately 2 pounds

1 Tablespoon olive oil

2 Tablespoons fresh rosemary, chopped

1 Tablespoon fresh thyme, chopped

Four garlic cloves, minced

One teaspoon dry oregano

One lemon, the zest

One teaspoon minced fresh ginger

1 cup (Good) red wine

Salt and pepper to taste

Directions:

Preheat the crockpot on low.

In a pan, heat one tablespoon olive oil. Brown the meat for 2 minutes per side.

Mix remaining ingredients in a bowl.

Place the lamb in the crockpot, pour the remaining seasoning over the meat.

Cover, cook on low for 8 hours.

Nutrition: Calories: 140 Carbs: 3g Fat: 5g Protein: 21g

CHAPTER 11:

Side Dish Recipes

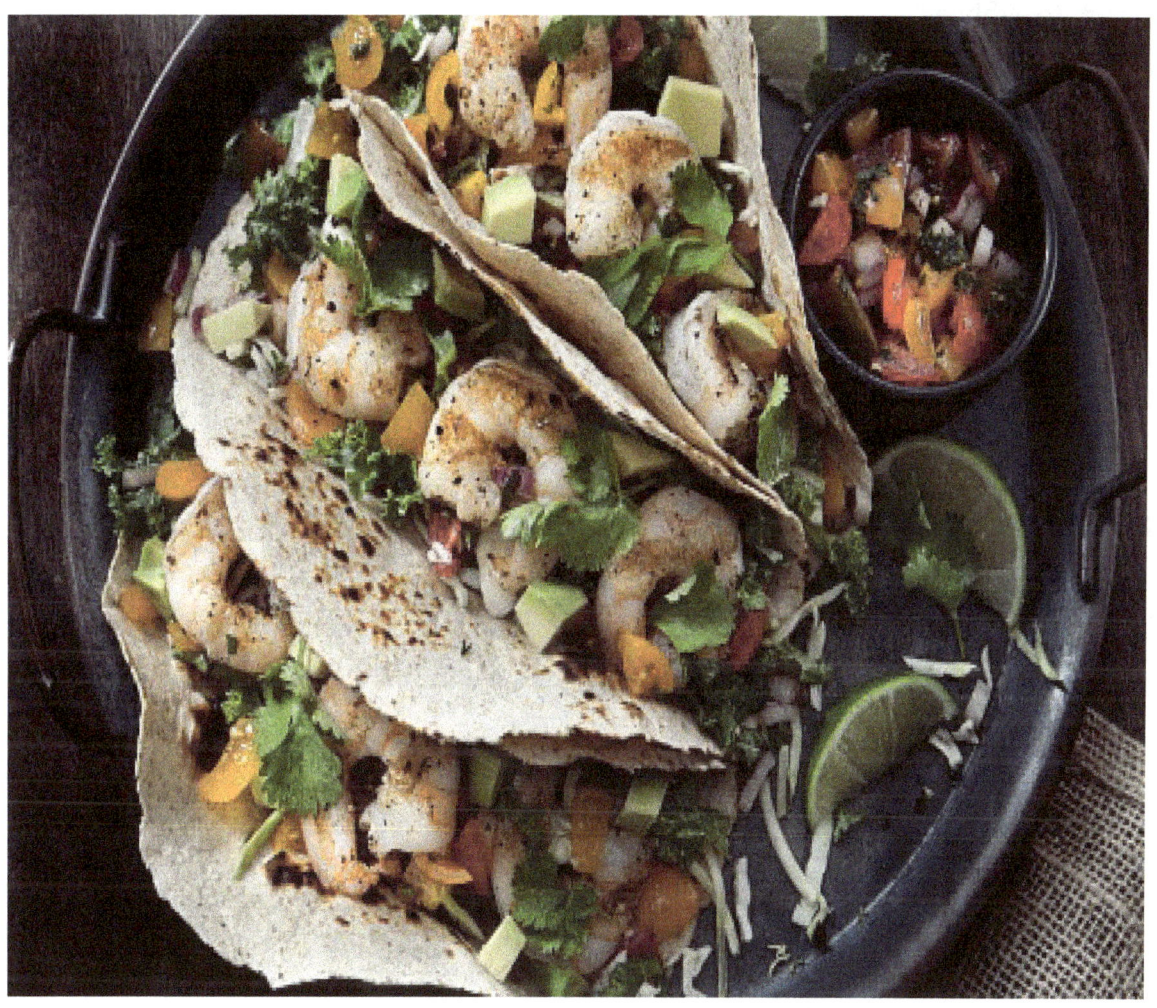

53. Cabbage Steaks

Preparation time: 15 minutes

Cooking time: 2 hours

Servings: 4

Ingredients:

10 oz white cabbage

One tablespoon butter

½ teaspoon cayenne pepper

½ teaspoon chili flakes

Four tablespoons water

Directions:

Slice the cabbage into medium steaks and rub them with the cayenne pepper and chili flakes.

Rub the cabbage steaks with butter on each side.

Place them in the slow cooker and sprinkle with water.

Close the lid and cook the cabbage steaks for 2 hours on High.

When the cabbage steaks are cooked, they should be tender to the touch.

Serve the cabbage steak after 10 minutes of chilling.

Nutrition: Calories 44 Fat 3 Fiber 1.8 Carbs 4.3 Protein 1

54. Mashed Cauliflower

Preparation time: 20 minutes

Cooking time: 3 hours

Servings: 5

Ingredients:

Three tablespoons butter

1-pound cauliflower

One tablespoon full-fat cream

One teaspoon salt

One teaspoon ground black pepper

1 oz dill, chopped

Directions:

Wash the cauliflower and chop it.

Place the chopped cauliflower in the slow cooker.

Add butter and full-fat cream.

Add salt and ground black pepper.

Stir the mixture and close the lid.

Cook the cauliflower for 3 hours on High.

When the cauliflower is cooked, transfer it to a blender and blend until smooth.

Place the smooth cauliflower in a bowl and mix it with the chopped dill.

Stir it well and serve!

Nutrition: Calories 101 Fat 7.4 Fiber 3.2 Carbs 8.3 Protein 3.1

55. Bacon-Wrapped Cauliflower

Preparation time: 15 minutes

Cooking time: 7 hours

Servings: 4

Ingredients:

11 oz cauliflower head

3 oz bacon, sliced

One teaspoon salt

One teaspoon cayenne pepper

1 oz butter, softened

¾ cup of water

Directions:

Sprinkle the cauliflower head with the salt and cayenne pepper, then rub with butter.

Wrap the cauliflower head in the sliced bacon and secure with toothpicks.

Pour water into the slow cooker and add the wrapped cauliflower head.

Cook the cauliflower head for 7 hours on Low.

Then let the cooked cauliflower head cool for 10 minutes.

Serve it!

Nutrition: Calories 187 Fat 14.8 Fiber 2.1 Carbs 4.7 Protein 9.5

56. Cauliflower Casserole

Preparation time: 15 minutes

Cooking time: 7 hours

Servings: 5

Ingredients:

Two tomatoes, chopped

11 oz cauliflower chopped

5 oz broccoli, chopped

1 cup of water

One teaspoon salt

One tablespoon butter

5 oz white mushrooms, chopped

One teaspoon chili flakes

Directions:

Mix the water, salt, and chili flakes.

Place the butter in the slow cooker.

Add a layer of the chopped cauliflower.

Add the layer of broccoli and tomatoes.

Add the mushrooms and pat down the mix to flatten.

Add the water and close the lid.

Cook the casserole for 7 hours on Low.

Cool the casserole to room temperature and serve!

Nutrition: Calories 61 Fat 2.6 Fiber 3.2 Carbs 8.1 Protein 3.4

57. Cauliflower Rice

Preparation time: 15 minutes

Cooking time: 2 hours

Servings: 5

Ingredients:

1-pound cauliflower

One teaspoon salt

One tablespoon turmeric

One tablespoon butter

¾ cup of water

Directions:

Chop the cauliflower into tiny pieces to make cauliflower rice. You can also pulse in a food processor to get refined grains of 'rice.'

Place the cauliflower rice in the slow cooker.

Add salt, turmeric, and water.

Stir gently and close the lid.

Cook the cauliflower rice for 2 hours on High.

Strain the cauliflower rice and transfer it to a bowl.

Add butter and stir gently.

Serve it!

Nutrition: Calories 48 Fat 2.5 Fiber 2.6 Carbs 5.7 Protein 1.9

58. Curry Cauliflower

Preparation time: 15 minutes

Cooking time: 5 hours

Servings: 2

Ingredients:

10 oz cauliflower

1 teaspoon curry paste

1 teaspoon curry powder

½ teaspoon dried cilantro

1 oz butter

¾ cup water

¼ cup chicken stock

Directions:

Chop the cauliflower roughly and sprinkle it with the curry powder and dried cilantro.

Place the chopped cauliflower in the slow cooker.

Mix the curry paste with the water.

Add chicken stock and transfer the liquid to the slow cooker.

Add butter and close the lid.

Cook the cauliflower for 5 hours on Low.

Strain ½ of the liquid off and discard. Transfer the cauliflower to serving bowls.

Serve it!

Nutrition: Calories 158 Fat 13.3 Fiber 3.9 Carbs 8.9 Protein 3.3

59. Garlic Cauliflower Steaks

Preparation time: 15 minutes

Cooking time: 3 hours

Servings: 4

Ingredients:

14 oz cauliflower head

One teaspoon minced garlic

Four tablespoons butter

Four tablespoons water

One teaspoon paprika

Directions:

Wash the cauliflower head carefully and slice it into the medium steaks.

Mix up together the butter, minced garlic, and paprika.

Rub the cauliflower steaks with the butter mixture.

Pour the water into the slow cooker.

Add the cauliflower steaks and close the lid.

Cook the vegetables for 3 hours on High.

Transfer the cooked cauliflower steaks to a platter and serve them immediately!

Nutrition: Calories 129 Fat 11.7 Fiber 2.7 Carbs 5.8 Protein 2.2

60. Zucchini Gratin

Preparation time: 10 minutes

Cooking time: 5 hours

Servings: 3

Ingredients:

One zucchini, sliced

3 oz Parmesan, grated

One teaspoon ground black pepper

One tablespoon butter

½ cup almond milk

Directions:

Sprinkle the sliced zucchini with the ground black pepper.

Chop the butter and place it in the slow cooker.

Transfer the sliced zucchini to the slow cooker to make the bottom layer.

Add the almond milk.

Sprinkle the zucchini with the grated cheese and close the lid.

Cook the gratin for 5 hours on Low.

Then let the gratin cool until room temperature.

Serve it!

Nutrition: Calories 229 Fat 19.6 Fiber 1.8 Carbs 5.9 Protein 10.9

61. Eggplant Gratin

Preparation time: 15 minutes

Cooking time: 5 hours

Servings: 7

Ingredients:

One tablespoon butter

One teaspoon minced garlic

Two eggplants, chopped

One teaspoon salt

One tablespoon dried parsley

4 oz Parmesan, grated

Four tablespoons water

One teaspoon chili flakes

Directions:

Mix the dried parsley, chili flakes, and salt.

Sprinkle the chopped eggplants with the spice mixture and stir well.

Place the eggplants in the slow cooker.

Add the water and minced garlic.

Add the butter and sprinkle with the grated Parmesan.

Close the lid and cook the gratin for 5 hours on Low.

Open the lid and cool the gratin for 10 minutes.

Serve it.

Nutrition: Calories 107 Fat 5.4 Fiber 5.6 Carbs 10 Protein 6.8

62. Moroccan Eggplant Mash

Preparation time: 15 minutes

Cooking time: 7 hours

Servings: 4

Ingredients:

1 eggplant, peeled

1 jalapeno pepper

1 teaspoon curry powder

½ teaspoon salt

1 teaspoon paprika

¾ teaspoon ground nutmeg

2 tablespoons butter

¾ cup almond milk

1 teaspoon dried dill

Directions:

Chop the eggplant into small pieces.

Place the eggplant in the slow cooker.

Chop the jalapeno pepper and combine it with the eggplant.

Then sprinkle the vegetables with the curry powder, salt, paprika, ground nutmeg, and dried dill.

Add almond milk and butter.

Close the lid and cook the vegetables for 7 hours on Low. Cool the vegetables and then blend them until smooth with a hand blender.

Transfer the cooked eggplant mash into the bowls and serve!

Nutrition: Calories 190 Fat 17 Fiber 5.6 Carbs 10 Protein 2.5

63. Sautéed Bell Peppers

Preparation time: 15 minutes

Cooking time: 5 hours

Servings: 6

Ingredients:

8 oz bell peppers

7 oz cauliflower, chopped

2 oz bacon, chopped

One teaspoon salt

One teaspoon ground black pepper

¾ cup coconut milk, unsweetened

One teaspoon butter

One teaspoon thyme

One onion, diced

One teaspoon turmeric

Directions:

Remove the seeds from the bell peppers and chop them roughly.

Place the bell peppers, cauliflower, and bacon in the slow cooker.

Add the salt, ground black pepper, coconut milk, butter, milk, and thyme.

Stir well, then add the diced onion.

Add the turmeric and stir the mixture.

Close the lid and cook 5 hours on Low.

When the meal is cooked, let it chill for 10 minutes and serve it!

Nutrition: Calories 195 Fat 12.2 Fiber 4.2 Carbs 13.1 Protein 6.7

64. Garlic Artichoke

Preparation time: 15 minutes

Cooking time: 2 hours

Servings: 4

Ingredients:

8 oz artichoke, trimmed, chopped

2 teaspoons butter

1 garlic clove, peeled

¼ cup water

½ teaspoon ground black pepper

Directions:

Chop the garlic clove.

Melt the butter and mix it with the chopped garlic.

Add the ground black pepper and stir the mixture.

Place the artichoke in the slow cooker and cover it with the butter mixture.

Add water and close the lid.

Cook the artichoke for 2 hours on High.

Transfer the cooked artichoke to a platter and serve!

Nutrition: Calories 45 Fat 2 Fiber 3.2 Carbs 6.4 Protein 2

65. Broccoli Stew

Preparation time: 15 minutes

Cooking time: 6 hours

Servings: 3

Ingredients:

6 oz broccoli, chopped

1 cup spinach

¾ cup almond milk, unsweetened

2 oz white cabbage, shredded

One tablespoon butter

One teaspoon salt

One teaspoon white pepper

2 cups of water

Directions:

Chop the spinach and place it in the slow cooker.

Add chopped broccoli, almond milk, shredded cabbage, butter, salt, water, and white pepper.

Stir the ingredients and close the lid.

Cook the stew for 6 hours on Low.

Stir the stew gently and transfer to serving bowls.

Enjoy!

Nutrition: Calories 200 Fat 18.4 Fiber 3.7 Carbs 9 Protein 3.6

CHAPTER 12:

Dessert Recipes

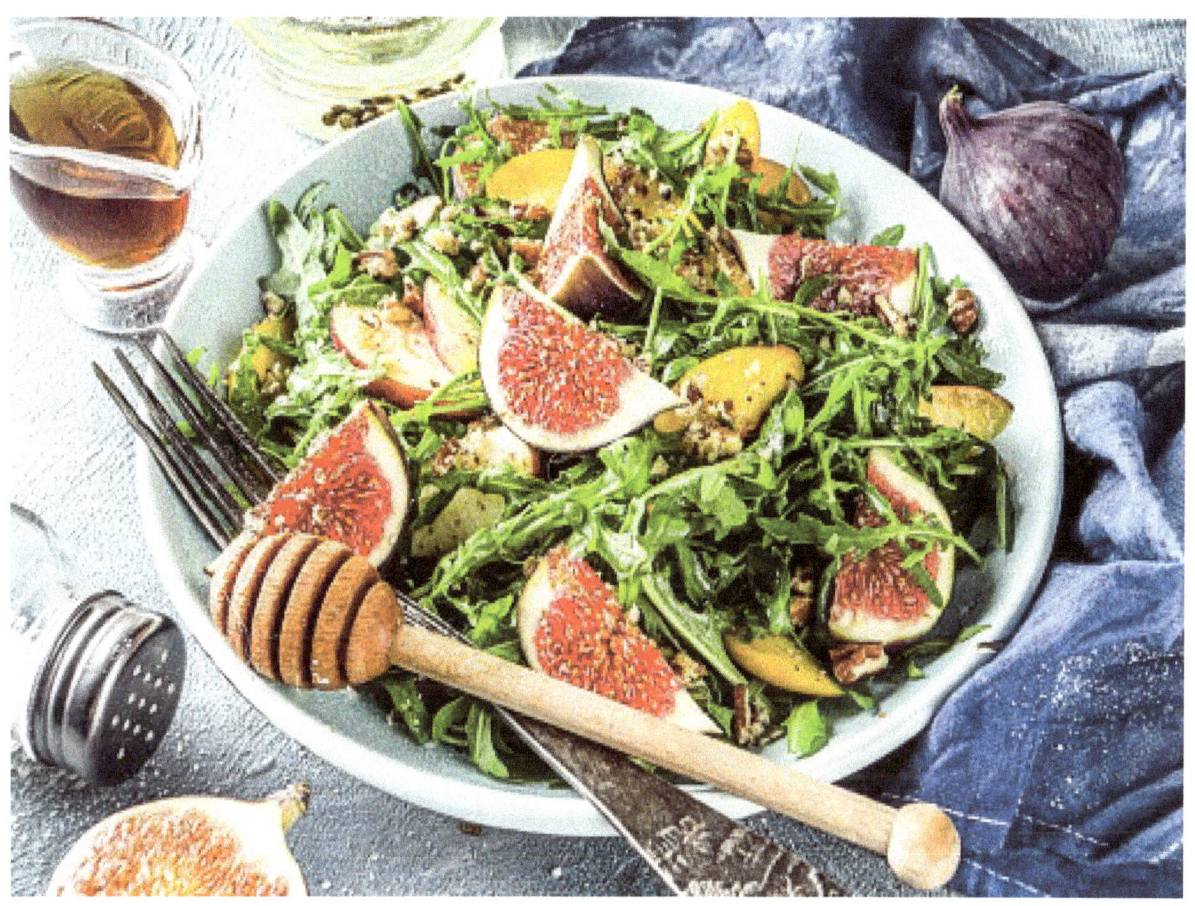

66. Tapioca and Chia Pudding

Preparation time: 10 minutes

Cooking time: 3 hours

Servings: 2

Ingredients:

1 cup almond milk - ¼ cup tapioca pearls

Two tablespoons chia seeds

Two eggs whisked

½ teaspoon vanilla extract

Three tablespoons sugar

½ tablespoon lemon zest, grated

Directions:

In your slow cooker, mix the tapioca pearls with the milk, eggs, and the other ingredients, whisk, put the lid on and cook on Low for 3 hours. Divide the pudding into bowls and serve cold.

Nutrition: Calories 180 Fat 3 Fiber 4 Carbs 12 Protein 4

67. Chocolate and Liquor Cream

Preparation time: 10 minutes

Cooking time: 2 hours

Servings: 4

Ingredients:

3.5 ounces crème Fraiche

3.5 ounces dark chocolate, cut into chunks1 teaspoon liquor

One teaspoon sugar

Directions:

In your slow cooker, mix crème Fraiche with chocolate, alcohol, and sugar, stir, cover, cook on Low for 2 hours, divide into bowls and serve cold

Nutrition: Calories 200 Fat 12 Fiber 4 Carbs 6 Protein 3

68. Dates and Rice Pudding

Preparation time: 10 minutes

Cooking time: 3 hours

Servings: 2

Ingredients:

1 cup dates, chopped

½ cup white rice

1 cup almond milk

Two tablespoons brown sugar

One teaspoon almond extract

Directions:

In your slow cooker, mix the rice with the milk and the other ingredients, whisk, put the lid on and cook on Low for 3 hours.

Divide the pudding into bowls and serve.

Nutrition: Calories 152 Fat 5 Fiber 2 Carb 6 Protein 3

69. Butternut Squash Sweet Mix

Preparation time: 10 minutes

Cooking time: 3 hours

Serving: 8

Ingredients:

2 pounds butternut squash, steamed, peeled, and mashed

Two eggs

1 cup milk

¾ cup maple syrup

One teaspoon cinnamon powder

½ teaspoon ginger powder

¼ teaspoon cloves, ground

One tablespoon cornstarch

Whipped cream for serving

Directions:

In a bowl, mix squash with maple syrup, milk, eggs, cinnamon, cornstarch, ginger, cloves, and cloves and stir very well.

Pour this into your slow cooker, cover, cook on Low for 2 hours, divide into cups and serve with whipped cream on top.

Nutrition: Calories 152 Fat 3 Fiber 4 Carbs 16 Protein 4

70. Almonds, Walnuts, and Mango Bowls

Preparation time: 10 minutes

Cooking time: 2 hours

Servings: 2

Ingredients:

1 cup walnuts, chopped

Two tablespoons almonds, chopped

1 cup mango, peeled and roughly cubed

1 cup heavy cream

½ teaspoon vanilla extract

One teaspoon almond extract

One tablespoon brown sugar

Directions:

In your slow cooker, mix the nuts with the mango, cream, and the other ingredients, toss, put the lid on and cook on High for 2 hours.

Divide the mix into bowls and serve.

Nutrition: Calories 220 Fat 4 Fiber 2 Carbs 4 Protein 6

71. Tapioca Pudding

Preparation time: 10 minutes

Cooking time: 1 hour

Servings: 6

Ingredients:

1 and ¼ cups milk

1/3 cup tapioca pearls, rinsed

½ cup water

½ cup sugar

Zest of ½ lemon

Directions:

In your slow cooker, mix tapioca with milk, sugar, water, and lemon zest, stir, cover, cook on Low for 1 hour, divide into cups and serve warm.

Nutrition: Calories 200 Fat 4 Fiber 2 Carbs 37 Protein 3

72. Berries Salad

Preparation time: 10 minutes

Cooking time: 1 hour

Servings: 2

Ingredients:

2 tablespoons brown sugar

1 tablespoon lime juice

1 tablespoon lime zest, grated

1 cup blueberries

½ cup cranberries

1 cup blackberries

1 cup strawberries

½ cup heavy cream

Directions:

In your slow cooker, mix the berries with the sugar and the other ingredients, toss, put the lid on and cook on High for 1 hour. Divide the mix into bowls and serve.

Nutrition: Calories 262 Fat 7 Fiber 2 Carbs 5 Protein 8

73. Fresh Cream Mix

Preparation time: 1 hour

Cooking time: 1 hour

Servings: 6

Ingredients:

2 cups fresh cream

One teaspoon cinnamon powder

Six egg yolks

Five tablespoons white sugar

Zest of 1 orange, grated

A pinch of nutmeg for serving

Four tablespoons sugar

2 cups of water

Directions:

In a bowl, mix cream, cinnamon, and orange zest and stir.

In another bowl, mix the egg yolks with white sugar and whisk well.

Add this over the cream, stir, strain, and divide into ramekins.

Put ramekins in your slow cooker, add 2 cups water to the slow cooker, cover, cook on Low for 1 hour, leave cream aside to cool down, and serve.

Nutrition: Calories 200 Fat 4 Fiber 5 Carbs 15 Protein 5

74. Pears and Apples Bowls

Preparation time: 10 minutes

Cooking time: 2 hours

Servings: 2

Ingredients:

One teaspoon vanilla extract

Two pears, cored and cut into wedges

Two apples, cored and cut into wedges

One tablespoon walnuts, chopped

Two tablespoons brown sugar

½ cup coconut cream

Directions:

In your slow cooker, mix the pears with the apples, nuts, and the other ingredients, toss, put the lid on and cook on Low for 2 hours. Divide the mix into bowls and serve cold.

Nutrition: Calories 120 Fat 2 Fiber 2 Carbs 4 Protein 3

75. Pears and Wine Sauce

Preparation time: 10 minutes

Cooking time: 1 hour

Servings: 6

Ingredients:

6 green pears

1 vanilla pod

1 cloves

A pinch of cinnamon

7 oz. sugar

1 glass red wine

Directions:

In your slow cooker, mix wine with sugar, vanilla, and cinnamon.

Add pears and clove, cover slow cooker and cook on High for 1 hour and 30 minutes.

Transfer pears to bowls and serve with the wine sauce all over.

Nutrition: Calories 162 Fat 4 Fiber 3 Carbs 6 Protein 3

76. Creamy Rhubarb and Plums Bowls

Preparation time: 10 minutes

Cooking time: 2 hours

Servings: 2

Ingredients:

1 cup plums, pitted and halved

1 cup rhubarb, sliced

1 cup coconut cream

½ teaspoon vanilla extract

½ cup of sugar

½ tablespoon lemon juice

One teaspoon almond extract

Directions:

In your slow cooker, mix the plums with the rhubarb, cream, and the other ingredients, toss, put the lid on and cook on High for 2 hours. Divide the mix into bowls and serve.

Nutrition: Calories 162 Fat 2 Fiber 2 Carbs 4 Protein 5

77. Pears and Grape Sauce

Preparation time: 10 minutes

Cooking time: 1 hour

Servings: 4

Ingredients:

Four pears

Juice and zest of 1 lemon

26 ounces grape juice

11 ounces currant jelly

Four garlic cloves

½ vanilla bean

Four peppercorns

Two rosemary springs

Directions:

Put the jelly, grape juice, lemon zest, lemon juice, vanilla, peppercorns, rosemary, pears in your slow cooker, cover, and cook on High for 1 hour 30 minutes.

Divide everything between plates and serve.

Nutrition: Calories 152 Fat 3 Fiber 5 Carbs 12 Protein 4

78. Greek Cream Cheese Pudding

Preparation time: 5 minutes

Cooking time: 2 hours

Servings: 2

Ingredients:

1 cup cream cheese, soft

½ cup Greek yogurt

Two eggs whisked

½ teaspoon baking soda

1 cup almonds, chopped

One tablespoon sugar

½ teaspoon almond extract

½ teaspoon cinnamon powder

Directions:

In your slow cooker, mix the cream cheese with the yogurt, eggs, and the other ingredients, whisk, put the lid on and cook on Low for 2 hours.

Divide the pudding into bowls and serve.

Nutrition: Calories 172 Fat 2 Fiber 3 Carbs 4 Protein 5

79. Rice Pudding

Preparation time: 10 minutes

Cooking time: 2 hours

Servings: 6

Ingredients:

1 tablespoon butter

7 ounces long grain rice

4 ounces water

16 ounces milk

3 ounces sugar

1 egg

1 tablespoon cream

1 teaspoon vanilla extract

Directions:

In your slow cooker, mix butter with rice, water, milk, sugar, egg, cream, and vanilla, stir, cover, and cook on High for 2 hours.

Stir pudding one more time, divide into bowls, and serve.

Nutrition: Calories 152 Fat 4 Fiber 4 Carbs 6 Protein 4

80. Greek Cream

Preparation time: 10 minutes

Cooking time: 1 hour

Servings: 2

Ingredients:

1 cup heavy cream

1 cup Greek yogurt

2 tablespoons brown sugar

½ teaspoon vanilla extract

½ teaspoon ginger powder

Directions:

In your slow cooker, mix the cream with the yogurt and the other ingredients, whisk, put the lid on and cook on High for 1 hour.

Divide the cream into bowls and serve cold.

Nutrition: Calories 200 Fat 5 Fiber 3 Carbs 4 Protein 5

CHAPTER 13:

7 Day Meal Plan

Day	Breakfast	Lunch	Dinner
1	Vanilla Pancakes	Braised Pork Belly	Creamy Keto Mash
2	Potato Breakfast Mix	BLT Chicken Salad	Pot Roast Beef Brisket
3	Breakfast Veggie Salad	Amazing Pulled Pork	Lamb Provencal
4	Breakfast Pizza Shrimp	Ginger Steak Broccoli	Whole Roasted Chicken
5	Pork Breakfast Sausages	Chili Verde	Cheesy Cauliflower Gratin
6	Veggie Turkey Smash	Meaty Cauliflower Lasagna	Pork Carnitas
7	Breakfast Sweet Pepper Hash	Lime Chicken with Savoy Cabbage	Creamy Ricotta Spaghetti Squash

Conclusion

When you shift to the ketogenic diet, it is essential to consider your overall health, and just like any eating plan, you need to maintain a healthy lifestyle to go with the diet. A healthy lifestyle is a choice. Just because we have thrown around the word "diet" does not mean that you should think of the ketogenic diet as something that only comes and goes. If you choose to use this dietary plan, you need to remember that you have to use it not necessarily for the rest of your life, but you will have to incorporate many healthier aspects for the rest of your life if you want to stay healthy. It takes diligence to do this, but it is well worth it. When you start living a healthier life, you may want to start small by changing your regular meal plan to one of the slow cooker ketogenic recipes each day. Slow changes like this can help you too, within one or two weeks, switch over without as much pressure. Eventually, you can turn all of your meals into approved ones, and if you miss a day or two, don't knock yourself up. Like anything you choose to do, this takes time before your body fully adjusts.

If your objective is losing weight and get healthy by using the ketogenic diet, remember that weight loss has to include exercise. Even if you cut carbs out almost entirely and follow every facet of the ketogenic diet, you still need to exercise. Make exercise a daily habit of your new lifestyle just the same as making the food you regularly take a daily part of your lifestyle. Doing so will maximize all of your weight loss results.

You need to know that your body will respond to the demand you put on it, and it will react to the Keto food changes and exercise with time. If you ask your muscles to lift something heavy, it will get stronger and lift something heavy. If you ask your muscles to stay stagnant and sit on the couch, they will shrivel up and do exactly that.

Exercise damages your muscle, which then allows your body to remodel the strength to prevent further injury. Each time you train the small fibers, you injure them and force them to get bigger and stronger. It means that intense exercise is essential.

Your muscles respond to calories. Research shows that people who restrict their calories end up losing muscle mass with slower digestion or metabolism. Essential calorie restriction is not enough. It is necessary that you eat and that you eat well and exercise simultaneously.

The proteins and the fluid in your muscle fibers are broken down and rebuilt approximately every 7 to 15 days. Training can change this by impacting the type of proteins and the amount of protein your body produces.

Energy from your fat stores can be released and stored inside your muscle tissue, but you need ample nutrients and patience as this process takes place. Eating right is always the best way to go, and so is eating enough. Weight loss without proper calorie consumption is not something you should aim for.

Your hormones respond to exercise, and how they impact your weight loss depends heavily on your nutritional status, the number of calories you are consuming. Eating 2800 calories of pizza is not the same as 2800 calories of lean salmon and broccoli.

Your muscles (the ones that will help you burn fat or stay healthy) respond to calories. Research shows that people who restrict their calories to lose weight lose muscle mass with a slower metabolism. Simple calorie restriction is not enough. Some people who use stricter calories and field exercise ended up fatter than where they started. It is essential that you eat and that you eat well. It cannot be stressed enough to enjoy lots of fats and lots of proteins with the keto diet. You cannot hope to generate the same amount of energy your body derives from simple carbohydrates if you do not make sure you are getting enough fat. Remember, fat is now your primary energy source, so it should constitute a large part of your diet.

That said, you can reduce your carbohydrates quickly and make the change fast, or you can do it slowly and make the change gradually. As an athlete who wants to build muscle mass or better tone your body, you need to work hard enough to burn off all the items included in the meal and make sure that you have high energy to complete your workouts. You don't want to starve your body. Remember, the key to this particular diet is to get as many fats as you can.

Naturally, the time you spent eating out versus cooking at home is bound to change. When they switch to healthier diets, most people find that it is simply easier to have complete control over what you eat. You can never really trust a strange company to offer things how you like it, nor can you be sure that they will have healthier choices. Eating out doesn't have to go away altogether, but the more you learn about the ketogenic diet, the more you can make wise choices when attending company dinners or birthday events. Look up restaurants ahead of time and find out which ones serve the ketogenic friendly dish or have something that you can convert into a ketogenic close item.

You found a multitude of recipes included in this guide for a specific reason. When you eat at home, want to add variety. The worst thing you can do is to eat the same dull thing day in and day out. It will cause you to get frustrated with the diet. There are so many things that you can make for your Slow Cooker dinners, and you can substitute any number of vegetables or different meats until you find something with which you are entirely satisfied. Refer to the list of approved slow cooker recipes included and see if you can't mix-and-match any number of nutritious items regularly.

CPSIA information can be obtained
at www.ICGtesting.com
Printed in the USA
LVHW062027120121
676319LV00002B/6